CHAIR YOGA FOR WEIGHT LOSS

A Collection of 50+ Low-Impact Exercises for Seniors and Beginners to Lose Weight While Sitting on a Chair. Includes Personal Trainer Video Tutorials and 28-Day Challenge

Claire Parker

TABLE OF CONTENTS

1. Neck Rolls **pag.8**	2. Shoulder Rolls **pag.9**	3. Wrist Circles **pag.10**	4. Seated Cat-Cow Stretch **pag.11**	5. Ankle Circles **pag.12**	6. Seated Forward Fold **pag.13**
7. Prayer Pose **pag.15**	8. Side Twist **pag.16**	9. Seated Fold Pose **pag.17**	10. Cobra Pose **pag.18**	11. Low Lunge **pag.19**	12. Hands Up **pag.20**
13. Pigeon Pose **pag.21**	14. Single-Leg Forward Bend **pag.22**	15. Sun Breath **pag.23**	16. High Lunge **pag.24**	17. Warrior I **pag.25**	18. Humble Warrior **pag.26**
19. Roll-Down, Roll-Up **pag.27**	20. Deep Side Stretch **pag.28**	21. Foot Flexor **pag.29**	22. Cowface Arms **pag.30**	23. Leg Extensions **pag.31**	24. Boat Pose **pag.32**

49. Five-Point Star **pag.60**	50. Downward Dog **pag.61**	51. Child's Pose **pag.62**	52. Cat Pose **pag.63**	53. Knee Squeeze **pag.64**

INTRODUCTION

"Anybody can breathe, therefore anybody can practice yoga."
- T.K.V. Desikachar

If you are reading these words and still unsure about chair yoga, rest assured that it is the right book for you, no matter your age, your physical level, or your mobility range. I share the sentiments of Desikachar, a yoga master who believed in making it relevant to everybody - people from all walks of life and with all types of abilities. Thus regardless of your state of being, this book is for you.

Chair yoga, as the name suggests, involves settling into yoga poses while seated on a chair or supported by one. It is a gentle form of traditional yoga and is absolutely revolutionary as it makes yoga accessible to all individuals. Even those with mobility issues, seniors, and beginners to yoga.

In a typical yoga session, the yoga sequence often includes standing and floor poses which may be difficult or even dangerous for individuals who have balance issues or those without the strength to stand up on their own. In a chair yoga session, these standing and floor poses are adapted to incorporate the stability of a chair and practitioners still reap the benefits of yoga. Therefore it is a practical and inclusive approach that allows people of all ages and abilities to experience yoga.

The timeless wisdom of yoga has always provided an illuminating path toward holistic well-being. Similarly, the gentle practice of chair yoga can bestow myriad benefits to consistent practitioners. In this book, one of my goals is to share with you these benefits, including its ability to support weight loss while improving both your physical and mental health. The first chapter of the book provides more information regarding these benefits.

My second goal is to provide you with pragmatic guidance on how to seamlessly integrate chair yoga into the cadence of your daily life. Are you a busy professional who finds difficulty carving time away from your desk? Or perhaps a senior who can no longer stand without support? This book will be packed with exercises, routines, and precautions that you can tailor fit to ensure your own suitable and safe progression.

Refer to our image index found at the beginning of the book anytime you need a quick visual reference to the adapted poses. Follow the step-by-step instructions in Chapter 2 to perform the individual poses to the best of your ability. Feel the inherent power and healing quality of your breath as you flow through Chapter 3. When you are ready to go further, attempt one of the illustrated workout routines found in Chapter 4.

The book is organized and structured to aid your progress. You can scan the accompanying QR codes provided to access videos of the poses and/or routines. These videos are value-building tools specially created and curated to help you solidify your somatic practices. If you cannot properly view the content of the QR codes, please email us at info@balancedlivingbooks.com and we will help you resolve the issue.

A GIFT FOR YOU

Finally, it is my wish that by the end of the book, through the practice of poses shared within these pages, you will be empowered, inspired, and motivated. May you be empowered to take charge and assume full responsibility for your health, inspired to keep up a daily chair yoga practice, and motivated to pursue your weight loss dream with confidence and determination.

Before You Begin

We value you and want to provide you with all the tools you need to maximize your weight loss efforts. Because of this, we've put together a gift pack to help accelerate your progress with chair yoga.

To access your gift that contains:

- Your audiobook
- Video files to download so you can work out offline
- Fitness tracker

Scan the QR code below. Alternatively, send us an email to info@balancedlivingbooks.com using the magic word **GIFT-CHAIR YOGA WEIGHT LOSS.**

CHAPTER 1:
THE BENEFITS OF CHAIR YOGA AND SETTING UP YOUR SPACE

Chair yoga offers a gentle yet effective way to experience the time-honored wisdom of yoga, regardless of your age, physical condition, or mobility level. Incorporating the stability and support of a chair makes the practice of yoga accessible to everyone, including seniors, people with limited mobility, and those who are trying yoga for the first time. Before we begin with how to set up a proper chair yoga space and the equipment you may want to include in your practice, let's take a look at the benefits of chair yoga.

We begin with the reason you're reading this book—weight loss. While seemingly simple, chair yoga has the ability to improve your physical health and aid in weight loss. As you move through the gentle, (but effective poses and flow of exercises), your body will become more flexible, strong, and balanced. These improvements not only gradually improve your overall fitness level but also help boost your metabolism and increase calorie burn. This of course means weight loss when supported by a nutrition-dense diet. It also means that with consistent practice, chair yoga can help you achieve and maintain a healthy weight, reducing the risk of chronic conditions like heart disease, diabetes, and high blood pressure.

For those of you with limited mobility or physical challenges, chair yoga offers an accessible and inclusive path to experiencing all of the benefits of yoga. In adapting traditional yoga poses to the support of a chair, you're able to build strength and stability without the need for equipment or professional assistance. This means yoga is suitable for everyone—all ages, all abilities, and all fitness levels!

Beyond the physical benefits of chair yoga, the practice helps to enhance your mental and psychological well-being. In a time when so much is changing for you and the world is plagued by stress and anxiety, the relaxation techniques, mindful breathing, and meditation elements of chair yoga help you calm your mind, reduce stress levels, and promote a greater sense of inner peace. Focusing on the present moment, connecting with your breath, and tuning into the sensations of your movements activates your parasympathetic nervous system—the system needed to recover from stress and build resilience over time.

Using chair yoga provides you with a unique opportunity for self-discovery and personal growth through self-reflection, a deeper understanding of your thoughts, and silencing your inner critic as you overcome more difficult poses. This can lead to heightened self-awareness, shifting your perspective to one that is self-empowering, confident, and capable.

Finally, getting involved in chair yoga provides you with a gateway for making wonderful connections to fellow practitioners and a special community of yoga enthusiasts around the world. This could mean practicing while using the videos supplied while others are joining you in doing the same thing, gathering together a group of friends to work out with, or joining a community center or a chair yoga group that shares your passion for self-care and personal growth. This sense of connection and belonging can be incredibly uplifting, providing encouragement, motivation, and a safe space to explore your practice.

As you continue to explore the world of chair yoga, you will discover countless other benefits. These advantages could extend to improved sleep and increased energy levels to enhanced creativity and a more positive outlook on life. Because the transformative power of chair yoga knows no bounds when you give it a chance to change your life.

1. Setting Up Your Space

Now that you know about the benefits of chair yoga, it is time to create an environment that will nurture your practice.

- The first step in designing your personal chair yoga sanctuary is to choose a quiet, clutter-free area where you have sufficient space to move freely without distractions. This space should be wide and high enough for you to perform standing poses without fear of injury, bumping into things, or feeling constricted. While not absolutely necessary, I would recommend some customization of your space so that you can fully immerse yourself in the present moment, leaving behind the worries and stresses of daily life. This could mean selecting a cozy corner of your living room, a peaceful spot in your bedroom, or even a tranquil outdoor location.

- With your space chosen, you can now begin turning it into your chair yoga sanctuary. You might want to consider soft, gentle light to create a calming ambiance for relaxation purposes. Lighting can be adapted by simply dimming your overheads, opting for the soothing glow of candles, incorporating salt lamps, or hanging up string lights. This subtle shift in lighting can help signal to your mind and body that it is time to unwind, release tension, and embrace the present moment.

- With lighting now taken care of, you will want to turn your attention to sensory elements that can complement your chair yoga experience. Take some time to put together a list of soothing background music, like gentle instrumental melodies or nature sounds. Consider engaging your sense of smell by diffusing essential oils or burning incense that will help promote relaxation and mental clarity—my favorite scents for yoga practice are lavender, peppermint, and sandalwood.

- Finally, as you personalize your chair yoga space, remember that it is a reflection of your unique self and preferences. Feel free to add meaningful touches that resonate with you. This could include inspiring artwork, photographs of loved ones, or treasured mementos. These personal elements can serve as gentle reminders of the intentions and motivations you've set for yourself and will boost your motivation on days when you're feeling low or demotivated.

Taking the time to mindfully set up your chair yoga space is not only about creating an inviting physical environment but also a loving act that says you're committed to a stronger, healthier life. So, as you settle into your chair and begin your practice, allow yourself to fully arrive in the present moment, knowing that you have created a safe and nurturing space to explore the power and capabilities of your body and mind.

2.   Necessary Equipment

While chair yoga requires minimal gear compared to other forms of exercise, having the right equipment can be the difference between comfortably moving through poses and workouts and your safety.

Of course, chair yoga requires a chair. You will need to select a chair that is sturdy, stable, and has a solid base to support you through each yoga pose. While some people prefer chairs with arm supports, I would suggest you opt for one without arms as this will allow for greater freedom of movement and flexibility.

In addition, you're going to need a chair with a straight back to help enforce proper posture and alignment in your seated poses. Chair with wheels must be avoided as they will compromise both your focus and your safety.

To further enhance the stability of your chair, you're going to need to position it on a non-slip surface. This surface can include a yoga mat or a carpet with grip—not a rug that can move. Chairs that are placed on unstable or sliding surfaces will cause you to focus on your equipment rather than on safely moving through each of your poses.

Next, you're going to want to wear comfortable clothing that allows you to move. Choose breathable, stretchy fabrics that will move with you as you flow through the poses. Having said that, you're going to want to avoid clothing that is too loose or baggy, as it may get in the way or cause distractions during your practice. Remember, your clothing should feel like a second skin, allowing you to focus fully on your breath, movement, and inner experience.

Finally, to further support your practice, you're going to want to consider investing in a few optional props. These include yoga blocks, straps, and blankets that can provide you with additional support, and enhance your overall yoga experience. For example, a yoga block can be used to bring the ground closer to you in seated forward bends, while a strap can help you extend your reach and deepen your stretches. If you're not keen on spending a lot of money on your practice, you can improvise this equipment, using a thick hardcover book as a yoga block or a rolled-up towel as a strap. Blankets can also be used to provide extra cushioning and support during seated poses or as a yoga strap to allow you greater reach during difficult-to-do poses.

As with any form of exercise, staying hydrated is absolutely critical. Keep a water bottle nearby and take sips (but don't drink a lot of water) during your session. This helps you replenish fluids and maintain optimal hydration without becoming nauseous from overconsumption of water. Listen to your body's thirst signals and honor them with mindful sips of water as an act of self-care and nourishment.

As you gather your chair yoga essentials, remember that the most important element you bring to your practice is your own presence and your commitment to showing up for yourself. Approach your practice with a willingness to explore your body's capabilities and curiosity about your poses. After all, showing up and trying is better than doing nothing at all.

3. Chair Yoga Safety

As you prepare to dive into the world of chair yoga, we must take a moment to discuss the importance of safety in your practice. You cannot build a strong and stable foundation for your practice without prioritizing safety so that you can flourish and grow over the next few weeks. Observing safety precautions not only minimizes the risk of injury but also ensures that your chair yoga experience is a positive and enjoyable one.

Your safety only requires a few simple steps to care for your body and honor its unique needs, so let's look at some guidelines for your safety.

- One of the most important safety principles in chair yoga is to listen to your body and respect its limits. Your body is your wisest teacher, and it will always guide you toward what is safe, healthy, and appropriate for you in each moment. Pay close attention to your body's sensations and any signs of discomfort or pain and do not continue with your pose if you feel these. This is how your body is communicating to you that something is off and that you need to readjust, include props, or revisit a pose when your body is stronger and more flexible.

- While honoring your body's signals, be compassionate and understand that it is perfectly acceptable to modify your poses. Chair yoga is not meant to push you to your limits or promote perfection. Instead, it is about meeting yourself exactly where you are and celebrating the unique beauty and strength of your own body in a specific moment. One way to ensure that your practice remains safe and accessible is to use props or variations to modify poses as needed. If a pose feels too intense, use that yoga block, strap, or blanket to provide additional support or to help you find a more appropriate alignment. Remember, there is no shame in modifying a pose to suit your needs. In fact, doing so is a powerful act of self-care and self-respect.

- As you move through your chair yoga practice, it is also important to pay attention to proper alignment and technique. This means engaging your core muscles, maintaining good posture, and moving mindfully through each pose. Proper alignment and breath ensure you are getting the most out of each movement. If you are unsure about how to properly align yourself in a particular pose, do not hesitate to consult the illustrations and videos provided in this book so that you can readjust your body and include any props you may need.

- Finally, if you have any pre-existing medical conditions or concerns, it is always a good idea to consult with a healthcare professional before starting a new exercise regimen, including chair yoga. Your healthcare provider can offer personalized guidance and recommendations to help you practice safely and effectively, taking into account your unique health history and needs.

Remember, your chair yoga practice is a personal journey, and your space and practice should evolve and adapt alongside you. Feel free to experiment with different elements and arrangements until you find a setup that truly resonates with your needs and intentions.

CHAPTER 2:
STEP-BY-STEP INSTRUCTIONS FOR CHAIR YOGA POSES

Before you begin your chair yoga workouts, it's important that you understand each of the required movements and how to perform these correctly. Below, you'll find each of the poses that make up your workouts. These poses are broken down into step-by-step instructions, an illustration provided, and an accompanying QR supplied for you to scan. After scanning this code, you will be directed to a short video clip, showing you how to complete your poses and movements with the proper posture, alignment, and breathwork.

WARM-UP EXERCISES

Warming up is absolutely essential to help prepare your body for the upcoming chair yoga poses. The warm-up exercises below are designed to help increase blood circulation to lubricate your muscles and joints and help you prevent injury. Furthermore, proper warm-ups ensure you are firing up your metabolism before your workout even begins, aiding in more efficient weight loss.

TRAIN OFFLINE

Remember that your gift pack includes video files of all your poses. Download these videos to your computer so you can work offline, eliminating the need to scan each pose with your mobile phone. You can access your free gift by scanning the QR code in the introduction of this book.

1. NECK ROLLS

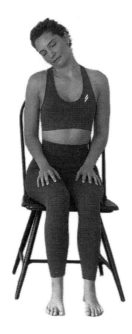
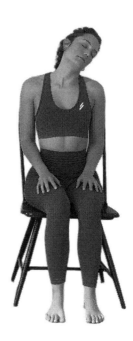

INSTRUCTIONS:

- Sit comfortably in your chair with your feet flat on the floor, and your hands resting on your thighs.
- Inhale deeply, and as you exhale, slowly lower your chin towards your chest, feeling a gentle stretch in the back of your neck.
- Begin to roll your head slowly to the right, bringing your right ear towards your right shoulder. Inhale as you roll.
- Continue the circular motion, bringing your head back, then to the left, and finally back to the center, completing one full circle.
- Repeat the motion, this time starting with your left ear towards your left shoulder.
- Perform 5-10 complete circles in each direction, moving slowly and with awareness.

GENERAL TIPS AND COMMON MISTAKES TO AVOID:

- If you experience any pain, dizziness, or discomfort during neck rolls, stop the movement immediately and return your head to a neutral position.
- Avoid rolling your neck too far back or pushing your chin too far forward. Keep your chin slightly tucked and limit the range of motion to a comfortable level.
- Avoid holding your breath or tensing your shoulder muscles during neck rolls. Remind yourself to relax your shoulders away from your ears and maintain a steady, natural breath pattern.

2. SHOULDER ROLLS

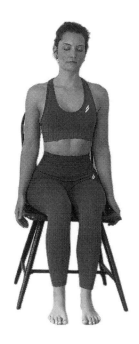 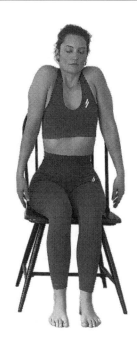

INSTRUCTIONS:

- Sit up tall with your feet flat on the floor and your hands resting on your thighs.
- Inhale deeply, then as you exhale, lift your shoulders towards your ears, squeezing them tightly.
- Begin to roll your shoulders back in a circular motion, moving them down, back, and then up towards your ears.
- Continue the circular motion for 5 to 10 repetitions.
- Reverse the direction of the shoulder rolls, moving them forward in a circular motion for another 5 to 10 repetitions.

GENERAL TIPS AND COMMON MISTAKES TO AVOID:

- Explore your full range of motion and use the largest comfortable circle as you do the shoulder rolls.
- Ensure the movement is targeted at the shoulders and avoid moving your elbows or arms excessively.

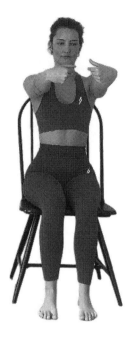 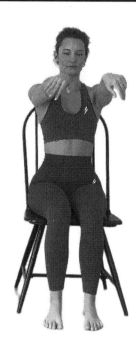

INSTRUCTIONS:

- Extend your arms out in front of you, palms facing down.
- Keep your hands relaxed, then begin to rotate your wrists in a circular motion.
- Perform 5 to 10 circles in one direction.
- Reverse the direction of the circles and perform another 5 to 10 circles.

GENERAL TIPS AND COMMON MISTAKES TO AVOID:

- Do isolate the movement to just the wrists and keep your arms and elbows straight during the exercise.

4. SEATED CAT-COW STRETCH

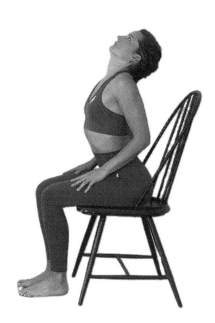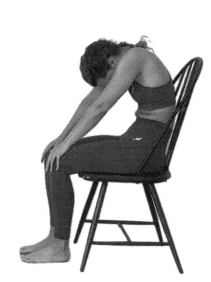

INSTRUCTIONS:

- Sit towards the front of your chair with your feet flat on the floor and your hands resting on your thighs.
- Inhale deeply, arch your back, lift your chest towards the ceiling, and gaze diagonally upwards (Cow Pose).
- Exhale as you round your spine, tucking your chin towards your chest and drawing your belly button towards your spine (Cat Pose).
- Repeat this flowing movement, coordinating your breath with the movement of your spine, for 5 to 10 repetitions.

GENERAL TIPS AND COMMON MISTAKES TO AVOID:

- Coordinate the movement with your breath.
- Slow down your breath and movement to maintain control and alignment.
- Initiate movement from the base of your spine up to your head.
- Avoid tensing the neck. Keep your neck relaxed, following the movement of your spine.

5. ANKLE CIRCLES

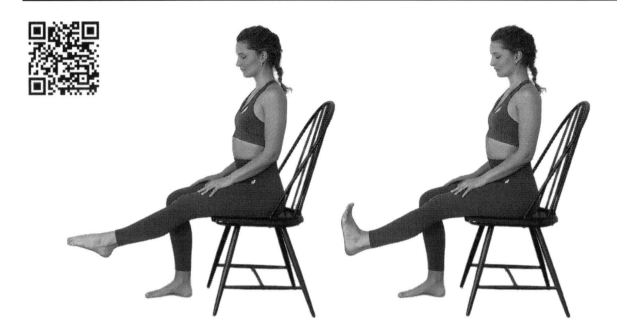

INSTRUCTIONS:
- Sit tall with your feet flat on the floor.
- Lift one foot off the floor and extend your leg in front of you.
- Begin to rotate your ankle in a circular motion, moving from your toes to your heel.
- Perform 5-10 circles in one direction.
- Reverse the direction of the circles and perform another 5-10 circles.
- Repeat the same steps with the other foot.

GENERAL TIPS AND COMMON MISTAKES TO AVOID:
- Do isolate the movement to just the ankles and keep your legs and knees straight during the exercise.

6. SEATED FORWARD FOLD

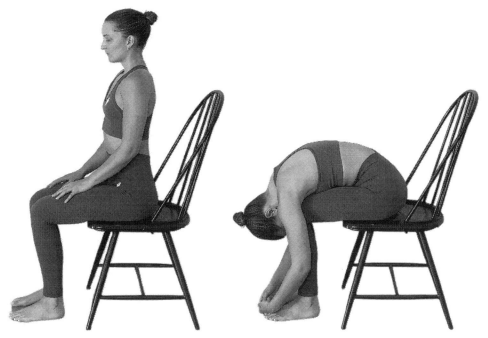

INSTRUCTIONS:

- Sit towards the front of your chair with your feet flat on the floor and your hands resting on your thighs.

- Inhale deeply and lengthen your spine.

- Exhale as you hinge forward at your hips, reaching your hands towards your feet or the floor.

- Allow your head to relax towards your knees, feeling a gentle stretch along your spine and the backs of your legs.

- Hold the forward fold for 20 seconds, breathing deeply and relaxing into the stretch.

- Inhale to slowly come back up to a seated position.

GENERAL TIPS AND COMMON MISTAKES TO AVOID:

- Let gravity do the work and totally relax when in the pose.

FULL BODY BASIC EXERCISES

These fundamental exercises adapt a range of traditional yoga asanas to be practiced safely and effectively with the support of a chair. They aim to awaken and mobilize your entire being. Each basic pose serves a crucial function, integrating flexibility, strength, and overall body awareness right from a stable seated position. Approach them with patience, proper form, and control of the breath. Recognize that these chair-assisted postures form the very foundation for unlocking yoga's multitude of benefits - from enhanced mobility and range of motion to more effortless movement patterns, to the metabolic boosts that aid natural weight regulation. Master the basics and the path to your fitness goals becomes clear.

7. PRAYER POSE

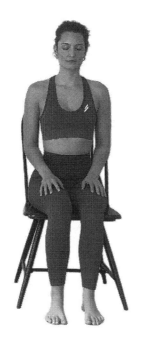 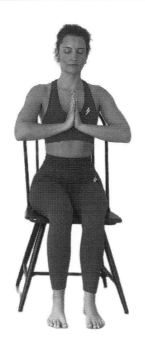

INSTRUCTIONS:

- Sit comfortably in your chair with your feet flat on the floor and your hands resting on your thighs.
- Take a moment to center yourself, closing your eyes if comfortable.
- Bring your palms together in front of your chest, fingers pointing upwards, in a prayer position.
- Press your palms firmly together and lift your chest slightly.
- Take a few deep breaths, feeling the connection between your hands and your heart.
- Hold the prayer pose for up to 20 seconds, focusing on your breath and setting an intention for your practice.

GENERAL TIPS AND COMMON MISTAKES TO AVOID:

- Avoid rounding your back or letting your shoulders slump forward. Keep your spine straight and shoulders back.
- Avoid lifting your shoulders towards your ears. Keep them relaxed and down.
- Avoid leaning forward, backward, or to the sides.
- Keep your head neutral and aligned with your spine. Avoid tilting or jutting your chin forward.

8. SIDE TWIST

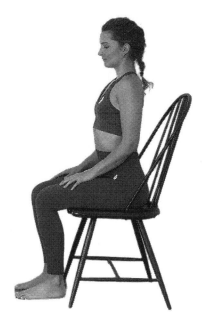
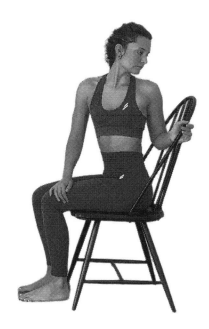

INSTRUCTIONS:

- Sit tall in your chair with your feet flat on the floor and your hands resting on your thighs.
- Inhale deeply and lengthen your spine.
- Exhale as you twist to the right, placing your left hand on the outside of your right thigh and your right hand on the back of the chair.
- Keep your spine tall as you twist, using your breath to deepen the stretch.
- Hold the twist for 10 seconds, breathing deeply and gently twisting a little further with each exhale.
- Inhale to come back to the center, then repeat the twist on the other side.

GENERAL TIPS AND COMMON MISTAKES TO AVOID:

- Ensure that your lower body remains square facing the front. Avoid over-twisting to the point that your knees and feet are out of alignment.

9. SEATED FOLD POSE

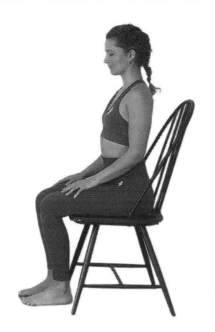

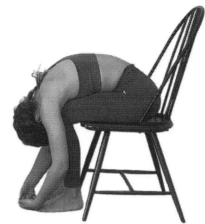

INSTRUCTIONS:

- Sit towards the front of your chair with your feet flat on the floor and your hands resting on your thighs.
- Inhale deeply and lengthen your spine.
- Exhale as you hinge forward at your hips, reaching your hands towards your feet or the floor.
- Allow your head to relax towards your knees, feeling a gentle stretch along your spine and the backs of your legs.
- Hold the forward fold for 20 seconds, breathing deeply and relaxing into the stretch.
- Inhale to slowly come back up to a seated position.

GENERAL TIPS AND COMMON MISTAKES TO AVOID:

- Let gravity do the work and totally relax when in the pose.

10. COBRA POSE

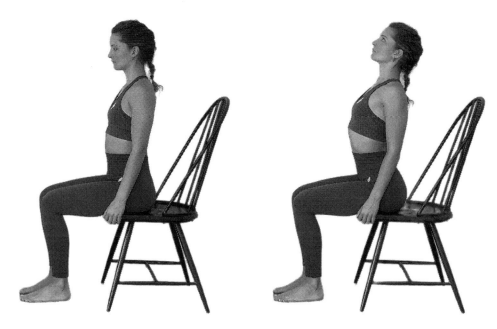

INSTRUCTIONS:

- Sit towards the front of your chair with your feet flat on the floor and your hands resting on your thighs.
- Inhale deeply and lengthen your spine.
- Exhale as you place your hands on the seat of the chair, slightly wider than shoulder-width apart.
- Press into your hands as you lift your chest and gaze upwards, arching your back gently.
- Keep your shoulders relaxed away from your ears and engage your core to support your lower back.
- Hold the cobra pose for 20 seconds, breathing deeply and enjoying the stretch through your chest and abdomen.
- Exhale as you slowly release back down to a seated position.

GENERAL TIPS AND COMMON MISTAKES TO AVOID:

- Avoid jutting your chin forward; keep your neck long and aligned with your spine.
- Keep your elbows close to your body; do not allow them to flare out.
- Ensure your feet remain flat on the floor for stability.

11. LOW LUNGE

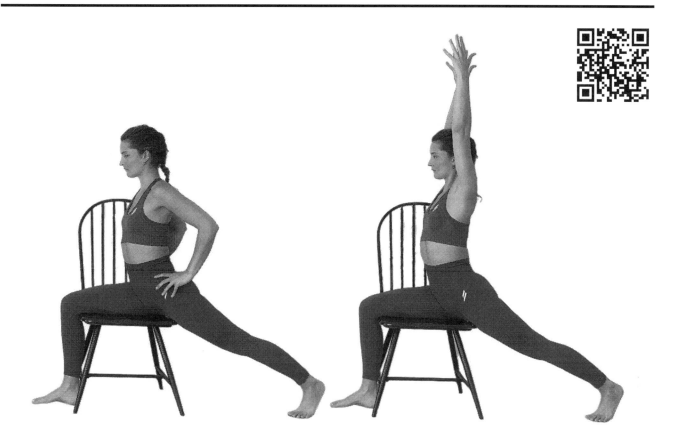

INSTRUCTIONS:

- Turn sideways in your chair with your feet flat on the floor.
- Extend your right leg behind you, placing the top of your foot on the floor.
- Keep your left foot planted firmly on the floor, with your knee directly above your ankle.
- Inhale as you lift your chest and engage your core.
- Exhale as you gently press your hips forward, feeling a stretch through the front of your right hip and thigh.
- Inhale once more and bring your hands up above your head in a sweeping motion, reaching for the ceiling.
- Hold the low lunge for 10 seconds, breathing deeply and sinking deeper into the stretch with each exhale.
- Inhale to release, then switch sides and repeat the stretch with your left leg extended behind you.

GENERAL TIPS AND COMMON MISTAKES TO AVOID:

- Position yourself so that your straight leg is in front of the chair and your bent knee is close to the seat of the chair to find the most stability.
- Change the direction you are facing when switching sides.
- To increase intensity, try to lift your body off the chair as you support yourself in the pose.

12. HANDS UP

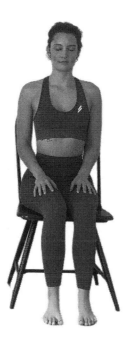
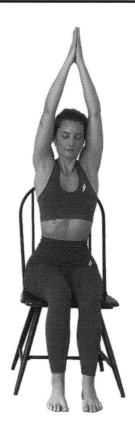

INSTRUCTIONS:

- Sit comfortably in your chair with your feet flat on the floor and your hands resting on your thighs.
- Inhale deeply and reach your arms overhead, bringing your palms together in a prayer position or keeping them shoulder-width apart with your fingers extended.
- Engage your core and lengthen your spine as you reach upwards, lifting your chest towards the ceiling.
- Keep your shoulders relaxed away from your ears.
- Hold the hands up position for 20 seconds, breathing deeply and stretching through your fingertips.
- Exhale as you slowly lower your arms back down to your sides.

GENERAL TIPS AND COMMON MISTAKES TO AVOID:

- Ensure that your weight is equally distributed on both sit bones throughout the exercise.

13. PIGEON POSE

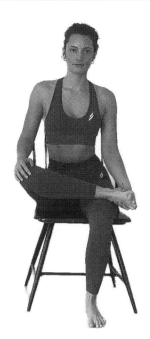 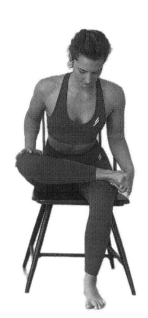

INSTRUCTIONS:

- Sit towards the front of your chair with your feet flat on the floor.
- Lift your right leg and cross your right ankle over your left thigh, flexing your right foot to protect your knee.
- Keep your left foot firmly planted on the floor.
- Inhale as you lengthen your spine, sitting up tall.
- Exhale as you gently hinge forward at your hips, keeping your back straight.
- You can use your hands for support on the chair or gently press on your right knee and ankle to deepen the stretch.
- Hold the pigeon pose for 10 seconds, breathing deeply and feeling the stretch in your right hip and glute.
- Inhale to slowly release, then switch sides and repeat the stretch with your left leg crossed over your right thigh.

GENERAL TIPS AND COMMON MISTAKES TO AVOID:

- Ensure that the ankle stays on the thigh and you are folding over the shin during the pose.

14. SINGLE-LEG FORWARD BEND

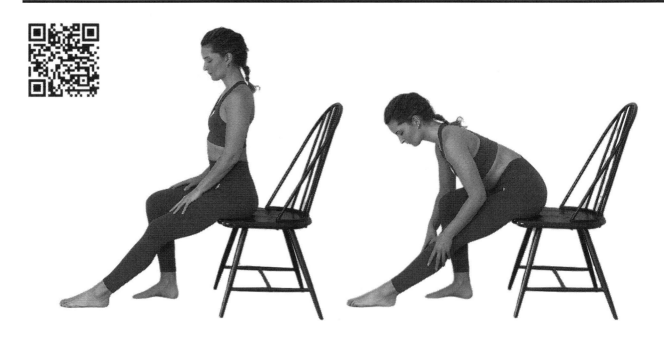

INSTRUCTIONS:

- Sit towards the front of your chair with your feet flat on the floor.
- Extend your right leg out in front of you, keeping your left foot planted on the floor.
- Inhale deeply and lengthen your spine.
- Exhale as you hinge forward at your hips, reaching your hands towards your right foot or ankle.
- Keep your back straight and your chest lifted as you fold forward.
- Hold the single-leg forward bend for 10 seconds, breathing deeply and feeling the stretch along the back of your right leg.
- Inhale to slowly come back up to a seated position, then switch sides and repeat the stretch with your left leg extended.

GENERAL TIPS AND COMMON MISTAKES TO AVOID:

- Do not lock your knee; keep a slight bend to avoid hyperextension.
- Avoid twisting your hips; keep them square and facing forward.
- Do not overstretch; move within your comfort zone and flexibility.
- Ensure your supporting foot remains flat on the floor for stability.

15. SUN BREATH

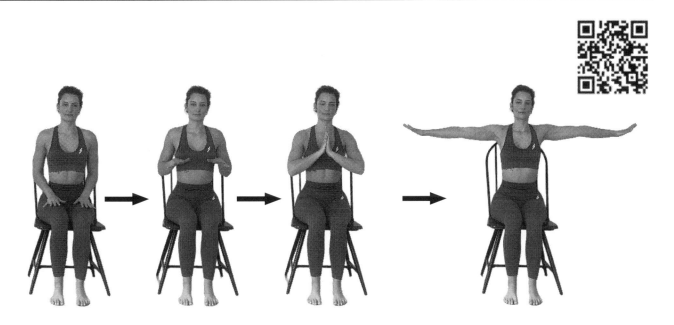

INSTRUCTIONS:

- Sit comfortably in your chair with your feet flat on the floor and your hands resting on your thighs.
- Place your hands palm down on your thighs.
- Inhale deeply as you raise your hands slightly above your thighs, keeping your palms facing down.
- Exhale slowly and bring your hands to the prayer position.
- Inhale deeply as you extend your arms out straight to your sides, palms facing the floor.
- Exhale slowly and bring your hands back to your thighs.
- This is one cycle.
- Complete 5 full sun cycles.

GENERAL TIPS AND COMMON MISTAKES TO AVOID:

- Coordinate the movement with your breath.
- Slow down your breath and movement to flow through the cycle smoothly.

16. HIGH LUNGE

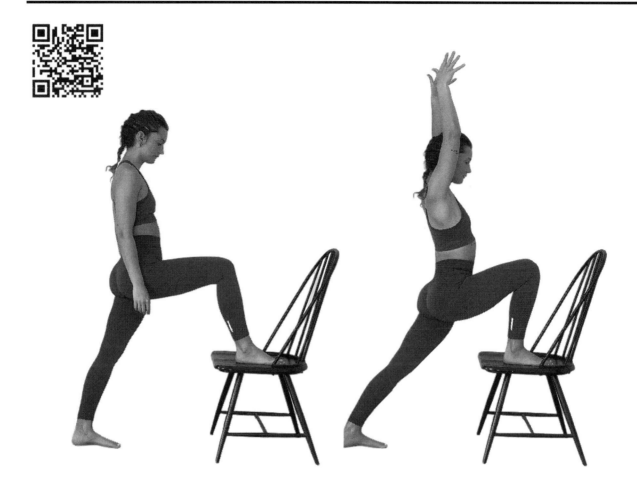

INSTRUCTIONS:

- Stand facing your chair's seat.
- Extend your right leg behind you.
- Keep your left foot planted firmly on the floor, with your knee directly above your ankle.
- Inhale deeply and lift your left foot, placing it on the seating area of your chair.
- Make sure your knee is stacked above your ankle.
- Place your hands on your thighs for balance or if you can, lift your arms up above your head.
- Exhale as you bend your left knee, sinking your hips down towards the floor.
- Keep your chest lifted and your shoulders relaxed away from your ears.
- Hold the high lunge for 10 seconds, breathing deeply and feeling the stretch through your left hip flexor and thigh.
- Inhale to release, then switch sides and repeat the stretch with your left leg extended behind you.

GENERAL TIPS AND COMMON MISTAKES TO AVOID:

- Depending on the height of your chair, you may need to adjust the placement of the extended leg to keep the bent knee directly stacked above the ankle.
- Maintain balance by keeping your center of gravity between your legs.

17. WARRIOR I

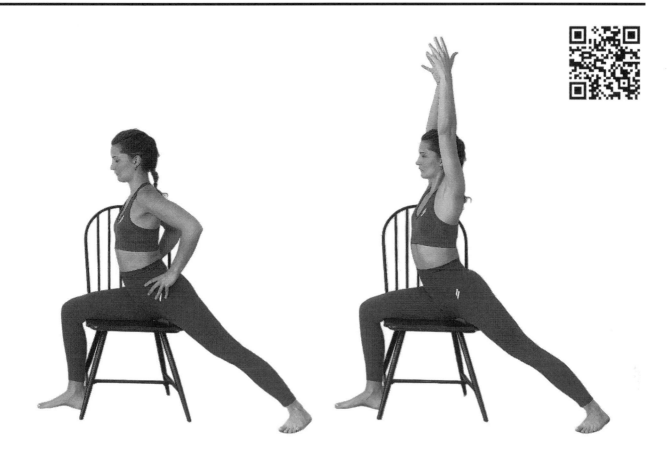

INSTRUCTIONS:

- Start by sitting towards the front edge of your chair with your feet flat on the ground.
- Extend your right leg back behind you, keeping your toes pointed forward and your heel lifted.
- Bend your left knee, ensuring it remains stacked over your left ankle.
- Inhale deeply as you raise your arms overhead, palms facing each other or touching.
- Gaze forward or up towards your hands.
- Hold the Warrior I pose for 20 seconds.
- Repeat on the opposite side, extending your left leg back and bending your right knee.

GENERAL TIPS AND COMMON MISTAKES TO AVOID:

- Position yourself so that your straight leg is in front of the chair and your bent knee is close to the seat of the chair to find the most stability.
- Change the direction you are facing when switching sides.
- To increase intensity, try to lift your body off the chair as you support yourself in the pose.

18. HUMBLE WARRIOR

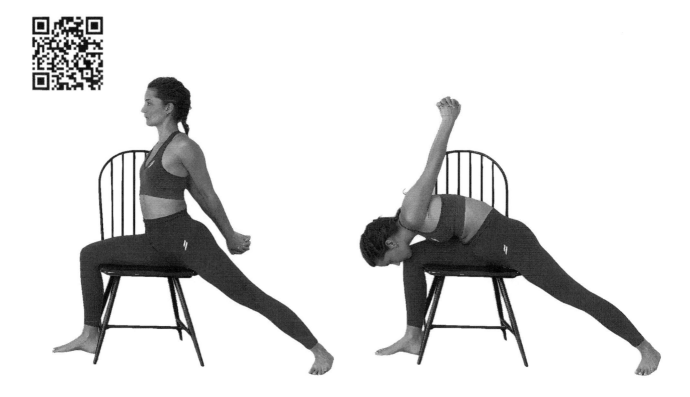

INSTRUCTIONS:

- Begin in the Warrior I pose, either on the right or left side.
- Interlace your fingers behind your back.
- Inhale deeply, then exhale as you fold forward from your hips, bringing your torso inside your front thigh.
- Allow your clasped hands to extend towards the sky as you maintain the interlace behind your back.
- Keep your back straight and your hips square.
- Hold the Humble Warrior pose for 10 seconds.
- Slowly release by straightening your front leg and returning to Warrior I.
- Repeat on the opposite side.

GENERAL TIPS AND COMMON MISTAKES TO AVOID:

- Position yourself such that the straight leg in front of the chair and the bent knee is close to the seat of the chair to find the most stability.
- Change the direction you are facing when switching sides.

19. ROLL-DOWN, ROLL-UP

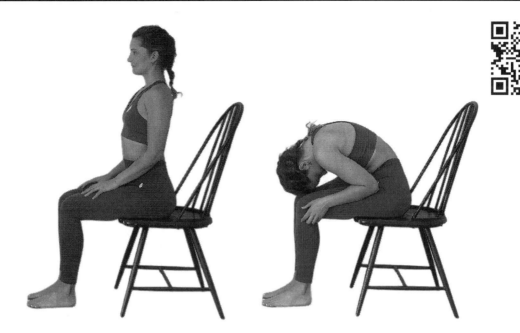

INSTRUCTIONS:

- Sit tall at the edge of your chair with your feet flat on the floor and your hands resting on your thighs.
- Inhale deeply and lengthen your spine.
- Exhale as you slowly tuck your chin to your chest and begin to roll down through your spine, one vertebra at a time.
- Keep your abdominals engaged and your movement controlled.
- Once you reach the bottom of your roll-down, pause for a moment, then inhale as you reverse the motion, rolling back up to a seated position.
- Repeat the roll-down, roll-up sequence 3 to 5 times, moving with your breath and focusing on articulating each vertebra.

GENERAL TIPS AND COMMON MISTAKES TO AVOID:

- Coordinate the movement with your breath.
- Slow down your breath and movement to flow through the cycle smoothly.

20. DEEP SIDE STRETCH

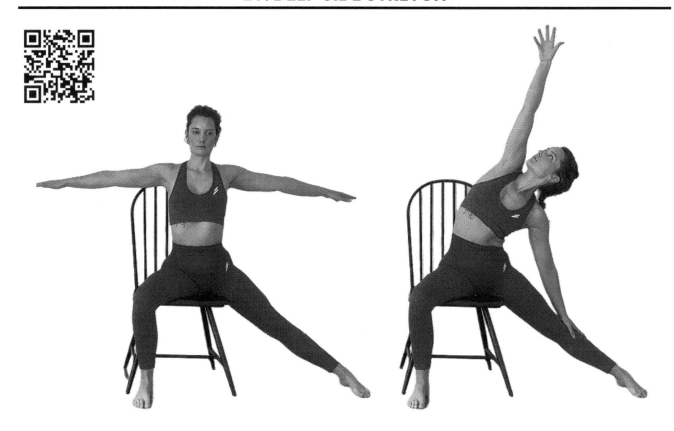

INSTRUCTIONS:

- Sit on your chair with your right hip close to the backrest.
- Extend your left leg out to the side, keeping it straight with your toes pointing forward or slightly angled upwards.
- Inhale as you raise your right arm overhead.
- Slide your left hand down your left leg as far as you can without bending your left leg.
- Exhale as you turn your gaze toward your right hand.
- Keep both hips grounded on the chair and avoid collapsing into the stretch.
- Hold the deep side stretch for 10 seconds, breathing deeply and feeling the stretch along your right side.
- Inhale to come back up to a seated position, then switch sides and repeat the stretch on the opposite side.

GENERAL TIPS AND COMMON MISTAKES TO AVOID:

- Ensure your hips remain stable and facing forward; don't let them twist.
- Do not overextend your arm; keep a slight bend in the elbow.
- Avoid tilting forward or backward; keep your torso in a straight line.
- Ensure the soles of both feet remain flat on the floor for stability.

21. FOOT FLEXOR

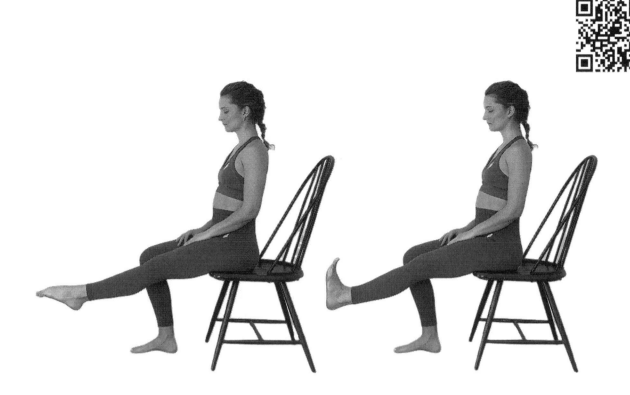

INSTRUCTIONS:

- Sit comfortably in your chair with your feet flat on the floor.
- Extend your right leg out in front of you. Lifting your foot off the floor.
- Keep your hands on your thighs and inhale as you flex your foot, pointing your toes up to the ceiling.
- Hold the flexed position for 5 seconds.
- Now point your foot, pointing your toes to the floor.
- Hold the pointed position for 5 seconds.
- Repeat with left leg extended.
- This is one full cycle.
- Complete 3 cycles.

GENERAL TIPS AND COMMON MISTAKES TO AVOID:

- Do not lock the knee of the extended leg; keep a slight bend to avoid hyperextension.
- To increase intensity, lift the extended leg higher to a 75-degree angle.

22. COWFACE ARMS

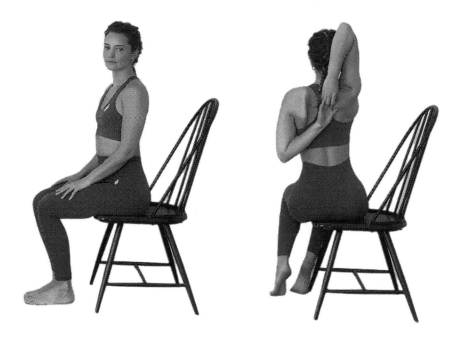

INSTRUCTIONS:

- Sit comfortably in your chair with your feet flat on the floor and your spine tall.
- Reach your right arm up towards the ceiling, then bend your elbow and let your right hand fall behind your head, palm facing your upper back.
- With your left hand, reach behind your back and bend your elbow, bringing your left hand up towards your right hand.
- Attempt to clasp your fingers together. If you can't reach your hands, you can hold onto a strap, towel, or shirt to bridge the gap between your hands.
- Once you've found your grip, gently draw your hands towards each other, feeling a stretch in your shoulders and chest.
- Keep your spine tall and your chest open as you hold the pose for 20-30 seconds, breathing deeply.
- Release the pose by slowly releasing your hands and bringing them back to your sides.
- Repeat the pose on the opposite side, reaching your left arm up and bending your left elbow behind your head, then reaching your right hand up to clasp your left hand behind your back.
- Hold the pose for 20-30 seconds on this side as well, breathing deeply and feeling the stretch.

GENERAL TIPS AND COMMON MISTAKES TO AVOID:

- Maintain a neutral head position by nudging your elbow back with your head if necessary.

23. LEG EXTENSIONS

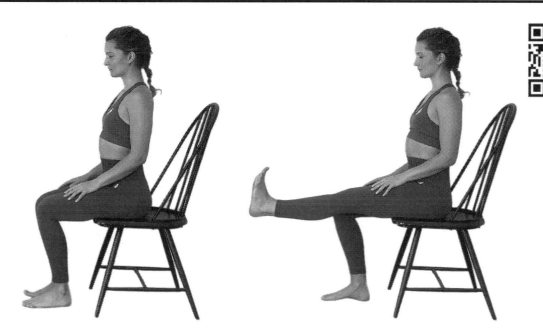

INSTRUCTIONS:

- Sit tall in your chair with your feet flat on the floor and your hands resting on your thighs.
- Extend your right leg forward, keeping your knee straight and your foot flexed.
- Hold the extension for a few seconds, engaging your thigh muscles.
- Slowly lower your right leg back down to the floor.
- Repeat the leg extension with your left leg.
- Continue alternating legs for 10 to 15 repetitions on each side.

GENERAL TIPS AND COMMON MISTAKES TO AVOID:

- Avoid swinging your leg; lift and lower it slowly and with control.
- Do not overextend your leg; move within your comfort zone and flexibility.
- Ensure your supporting foot remains flat on the floor for stability.
- To increase intensity, lift the extended leg higher to a 75-degree angle.

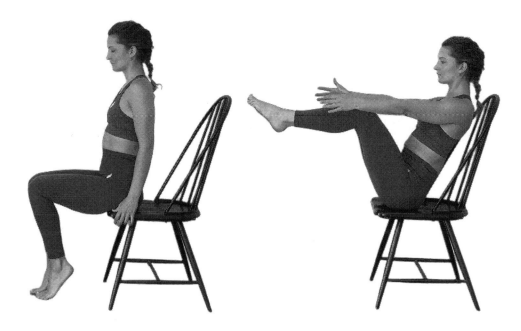

INSTRUCTIONS:

- Sit towards the front of your chair with your feet flat on the floor and your hands resting on your thighs.
- Inhale deeply and lift your feet off the floor, bringing your shins parallel to the floor.
- Extend your arms forward, parallel to the floor, palms facing each other.
- Engage your core muscles to maintain balance and stability.
- Hold the boat pose for 10 seconds, breathing deeply and keeping your spine straight.
- Release the pose with an exhale and lower your feet back down to the floor.

GENERAL TIPS AND COMMON MISTAKES TO AVOID:

- If necessary, start by leaning against the backseat and holding the seat of the chair with your hands.
- To increase intensity, try to straighten your legs such that your body forms a V-shape on the chair.

25. SAGE POSE

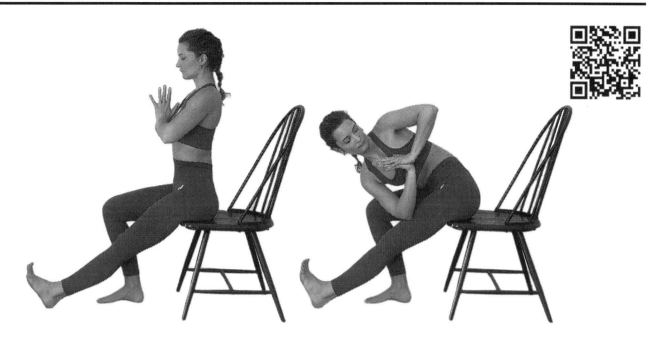

INSTRUCTIONS:

- Sit towards the front of your chair with your feet flat on the floor and your hands in prayer position.
- Extend your right leg straight out in front of you.
- Bend your left knee and place the sole of your left foot on the floor close to your right thigh.
- Inhale deeply and lengthen your spine.
- Exhale as you twist your torso towards the left, placing your right elbow on the outside of your left thigh.
- Press your elbow into your thigh to deepen the twist, and place your left hand on the back of the chair for support.
- Hold the sage pose for 20-30 seconds, breathing deeply and gently twisting a little further with each exhale.
- Inhale to release the twist, then switch sides and repeat the pose with your left leg extended.

GENERAL TIPS AND COMMON MISTAKES TO AVOID:

- Avoid collapsing the chest. Maintain a long spine in the twist.
- Ensure that both sit bones remain on the chair at all times.
- Press your palms together and bring them close to the heart center to deepen the twist.

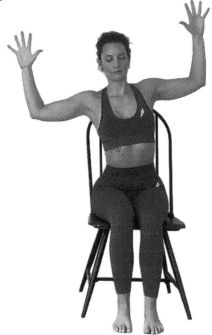 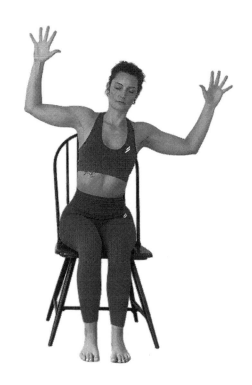

INSTRUCTIONS:

- Sit tall in your chair with your feet flat on the floor and your hands resting on your thighs.
- Extend your arms out to the sides at shoulder height, bending your elbows at 90-degree angles and spreading your fingers wide (resembling a cactus).
- Keep your shoulders relaxed away from your ears and your chest open.
- Hold the cactus arms position for 20 seconds, breathing deeply and feeling the stretch across your chest and shoulders.
- You can gently sway your upper body from side to side or lift your arms up and down to deepen the stretch.

GENERAL TIPS AND COMMON MISTAKES TO AVOID:

- Keep the arm muscles engaged and keep bringing the elbows away from each other.

27. REVOLVED POSE

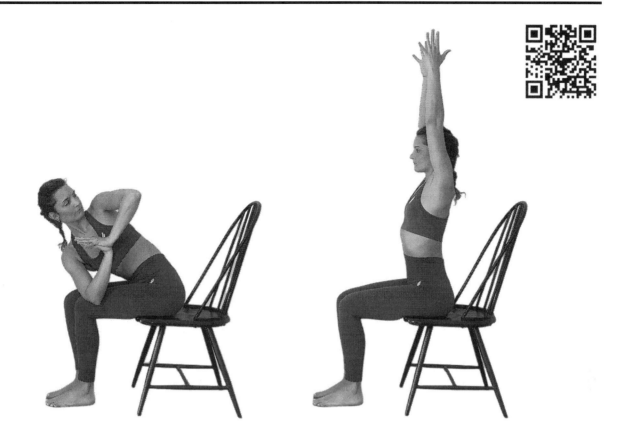

INSTRUCTIONS:

- Sit towards the front of your chair with your feet flat on the floor and your knees bent.
- Inhale as you lengthen your spine, lifting your arms overhead.
- Exhale as you twist to the right, bringing your left elbow to the outside of your right thigh.
- Press your palms together in a prayer position.
- Inhale to lengthen your spine even more, and exhale to deepen the twist, gazing over your right shoulder.
- Hold the revolved pose for 20-30 seconds, breathing deeply and feeling the twist through your spine.
- Inhale to come back to the center, then repeat the twist on the opposite side.

GENERAL TIPS AND COMMON MISTAKES TO AVOID:

- Press your palms together and bring them close to the heart center to deepen the twist.
- Ensure that the lower body remains square facing the front. Avoid over-twisting to the point that your knees and feet are out of alignment.

Muscle toning exercises are essential for strengthening and defining various muscle groups, promoting better balance, and enhancing overall functional fitness. This selection of exercises targets key areas of the body, focusing on both upper and lower body strength. Attack each rep with full focused engagement, squeezing the targeted muscles to their peak potential. Over time, this uncompromising approach amplifies muscular density and definition until your newly etched physique radiates power in repose.

28. SEATED LEG RAISES

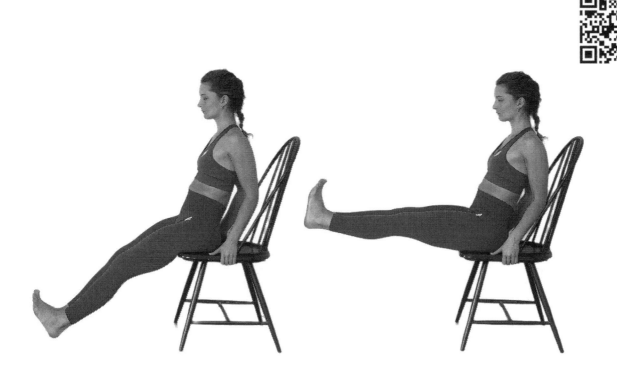

INSTRUCTIONS:

- Sit tall in your chair with your feet flat on the floor and your hands resting on your thighs.
- Lean back slightly on your seat.
- Place your hands on the side of the chairs at your hips for additional balance.
- Inhale as straighten your legs out in front of you.
- Exhale as you flex your feet with your toes pointed toward the ceiling.
- Inhale as you lift both of your feet off the floor, and hold your legs in this position for 3 breath counts.
- This is one repetition.
- Complete between 5 and 10 repetitions.

GENERAL TIPS AND COMMON MISTAKES TO AVOID:

- Avoid kicking your legs up; lift and lower them slowly and with control.
- Avoid swinging or tilting your upper body. Use your core and leg muscles to perform the exercise.
- To increase intensity, lift legs higher to a 75-degree angle.

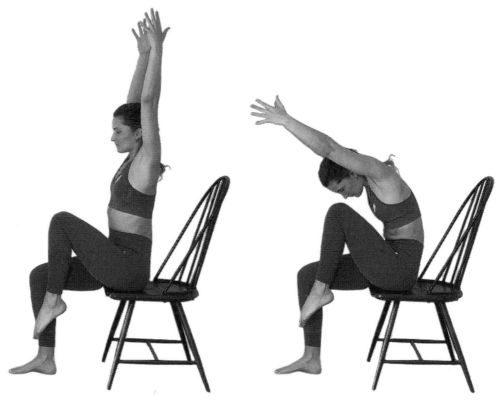

INSTRUCTIONS:

- Sit towards the front of your chair with your feet flat on the floor and your hands resting on your thighs.
- Inhale deeply and lift your right knee towards your chest.
- Exhale as you reach your hands up to the ceiling, arms straight and palms facing each other.
- Inhale and lean forward slightly, bringing your forehead towards your right knee.
- Hold the knee to nose position for 10 seconds, feeling the stretch in your upper back and shoulders.
- Inhale to release and return to an upright seated position.
- Repeat the knee to nose stretch with your left knee.

GENERAL TIPS AND COMMON MISTAKES TO AVOID:

- Expel the air from your belly fully to create space for your forehead to reach your knee.

30. CALF RAISES

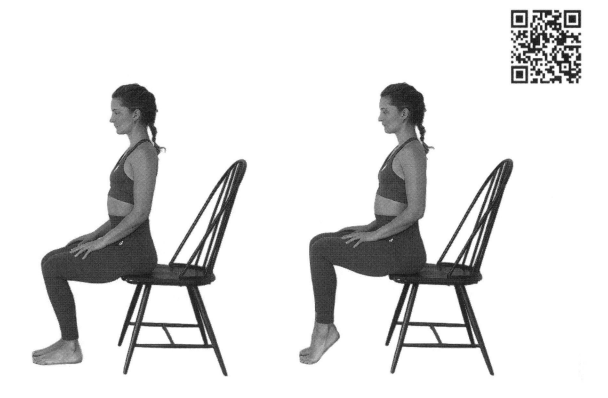

INSTRUCTIONS:

- Sit tall in your chair with your feet flat on the floor and your hands resting on your thighs.
- Inhale as you lift your heels off the floor, coming onto the balls of your feet.
- Exhale as you lower your heels back down to the floor.
- This is one repetition.
- Repeat this flow for 10 to 15 repetitions.

GENERAL TIPS AND COMMON MISTAKES TO AVOID:

- Lift and lower your heels slowly and with control; avoid sudden movements.
- Don't overextend your ankles; move within your comfort zone and flexibility.

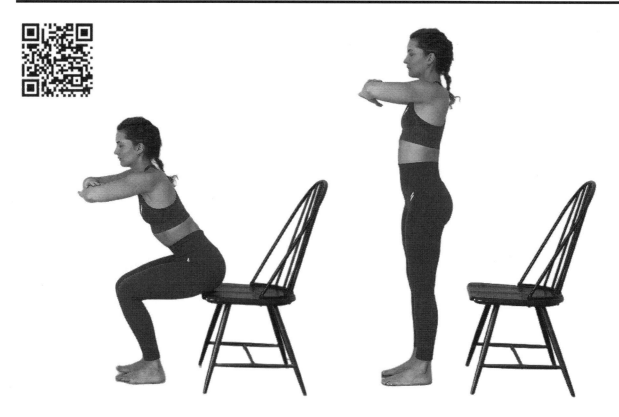

INSTRUCTIONS:

- Sit on your chair with your feet hip-width apart and your toes pointing forward.
- Bring your hands up to your chest, crossing them.
- Inhale deeply and engage your core muscles.
- Now, stand up.
- Keep your chest lifted and your weight in your heels.
- Exhale and lower down as far as is comfortable without ever sitting.
- Inhale as you press through your heels and straighten your legs to return to standing.
- Repeat the chair squats for 10 to 15 repetitions, moving slowly and with control.

GENERAL TIPS AND COMMON MISTAKES TO AVOID:

- Keep your spine straight and upright throughout the movement to prevent strain on your lower back.
- Ensure your knees stay in line with your toes and avoid letting them collapse inward or outward.
- Avoid using momentum to perform the squat; instead, focus on controlled movement.
- Keep the soles of both your feet flat on the floor throughout the movement to maintain stability and balance.
- Avoid locking out your knees at the top of the squat; keep a slight bend to maintain tension in your muscles.

32. SHUFFLE LEGS

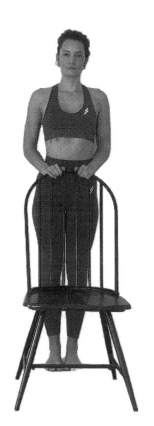

INSTRUCTIONS:

- Stand behind your chair facing the backrest.
- Place your hands on the backrest and stand up tall with a straight spine.
- Begin by lifting your right foot off the floor and tapping it lightly on the ground to the right side of your chair.
- Return your right foot to the starting position.
- Then, lift your left foot off the floor and tap it lightly on the ground to the left side of your chair.
- Continue alternating between tapping your feet to the right and left sides of your chair for 10 to 15 repetitions on each side.

GENERAL TIPS AND COMMON MISTAKES TO AVOID:

- Shift body weight fully to standing foot to lift opposite foot with ease.
- To increase intensity, lift your foot higher to a 45-degree angle before tapping it on the ground while keeping the leg straight.

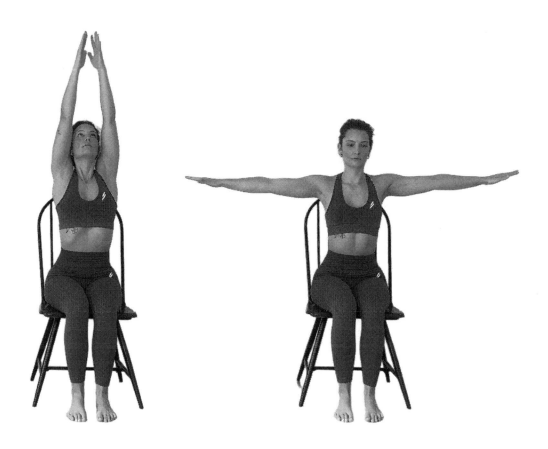

INSTRUCTIONS:

- Sit towards the front of your chair with your feet flat on the floor and your hands resting on your thighs.
- Inhale deeply and lengthen your spine, imagining yourself growing taller.
- Lift your arms overhead, reaching towards the sky, with your palms facing each other or touching.
- Keep your shoulders relaxed away from your ears and your gaze forward.
- Exhale and drop your arms to your sides, shoulder height with your palms facing down.
- Inhale and bring your arms down to rest at your side.
- This is one cycle.
- Complete up to 10 cycles.

GENERAL TIPS AND COMMON MISTAKES TO AVOID:

- Coordinate the movement with your breath.
- Slow down your breath and movement to flow through the cycle smoothly.

34. SINGLE-LEG CALF RAISES

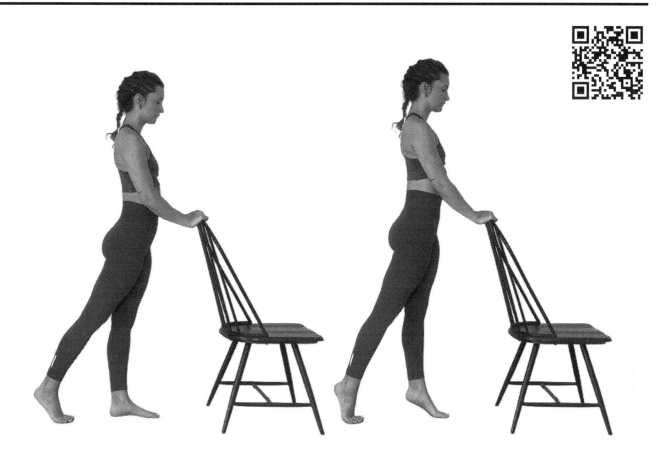

INSTRUCTIONS:

- Stand behind your chair facing the backrest.
- Place your hands on the backrest and open your legs about hip-width apart.
- Inhale, and extend your right foot slightly back, resting your foot on the ball.
- As you exhale, press through the ball of your left foot and lift your heel off the floor, coming onto your toes.
- Hold the calf raise for 5 seconds, then lower your heel back down to the floor.
- Repeat the calf raise with your left foot.
- Continue alternating between calf raises on each leg for 10-15 repetitions on each side.

GENERAL TIPS AND COMMON MISTAKES TO AVOID:

- Ensure that your body remains aligned throughout the exercise. Avoid leaning too far forward or backward. Keep your head, shoulders, and hips, in line with each other, maintaining a straight and upright posture.

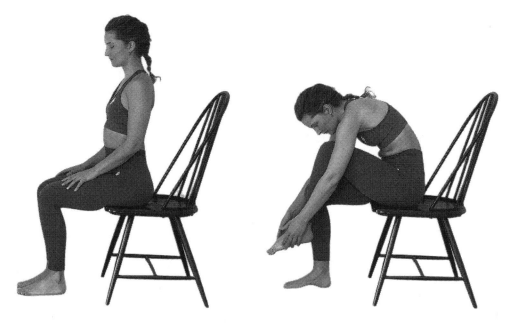

INSTRUCTIONS:

- Sit towards the front of your chair with your feet flat on the floor.
- Bring your hands up to lightly touch the back of your head with your elbows pointing outwards.
- Lift your right foot off the floor and reach your left hand forward to tap your right toes lightly—don't worry if you can't quite reach, tap the side of your right knee instead.
- Return your right foot and left hand to the starting position.
- Then, lift your left foot off the floor and tap your left toes or knees lightly with your right hand.
- Continue alternating between tapping your toes for 10 to 15 repetitions on each side.

GENERAL TIPS AND COMMON MISTAKES TO AVOID:

- Avoid bringing your knee too high; move within your comfort zone and flexibility.
- Avoid rounding your back; keep your spine long and straight.
- Avoid overtwisting. Hands and toes or knees should meet along the centerline of your body.

36. TRICEP DIPS

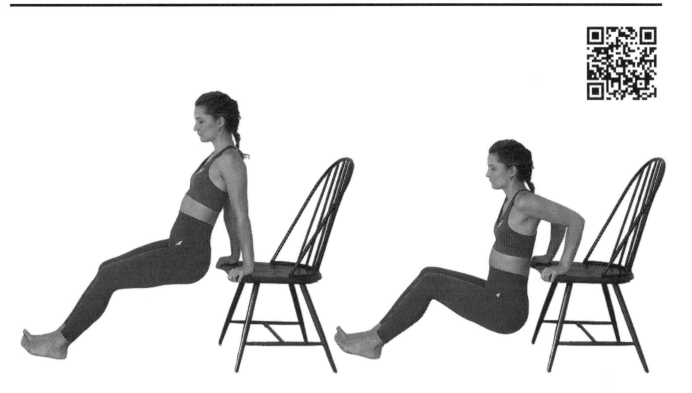

INSTRUCTIONS:

- Sit towards the front of your chair with your feet flat on the floor and your hands gripping the edge of the seat beside your hips.
- Slide your hips off the chair and walk your feet forward slightly.
- Inhale as you bend your elbows, lowering your hips towards the floor.
- Exhale as you straighten your arms, pressing back up to the starting position.
- This is one cycle.
- Repeat for 10 cycles.

GENERAL TIPS AND COMMON MISTAKES TO AVOID:

- Avoid overbending the elbows. Bend them only to a maximum of a 90-degree angle.
- Keep both feet flat on the floor.

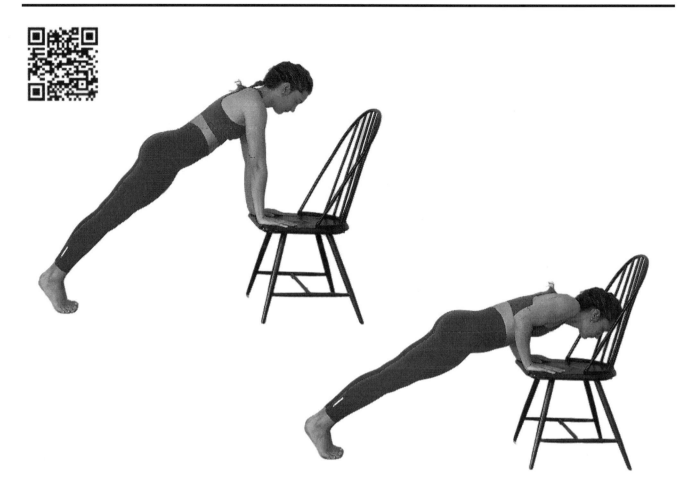

INSTRUCTIONS:

- Stand in front of your chair facing the seating area.
- Take a big step back and hinge at the hips bringing your hands onto the seating areas.
- Straighten your legs behind you.
- Now, inhale as you bend your elbows, lowering your chest towards the seat of the chair.
- Exhale as you press through your hands, straightening your arms and lifting your chest back up.
- This is one breath cycle.
- Complete for 10 cycles.

GENERAL TIPS AND COMMON MISTAKES TO AVOID:

- Always keep elbows close to your body.
- Maintain a straight line from head to heels.

FAT-BURNING EXERCISES

When it comes to igniting your body's calorie-burning furnace, these targeted exercises are your potent tools. Here you will find exercises that force your abdominal muscles to resist rotational forces or spike your core activation and metabolic expenditure. Your heart rate will rapidly elevate into prime fat-blasting zones. Perform these exercises with intensity and focus, squeezing maximum contraction out of every rep. Proper form enhances safety while amplifying the visceral fat-scorching effects. Consistency with these drills revolutionizes your body composition over time—stripping away stubborn fats while building up your muscles.

38. SEATED MARCHING

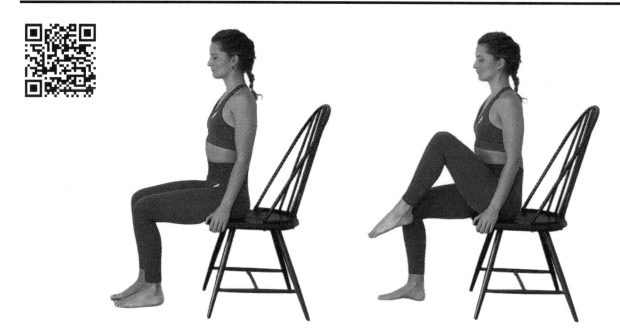

INSTRUCTIONS:

- Sit comfortably in your chair with your feet flat on the floor and your hands holding the seat of the chair for support.
- Exhale as you lift your right foot off the floor, bringing your knee towards your chest.
- Inhale and lower your right foot back down to the floor.
- Then exhale and lift your left foot off the floor, bringing your knee towards your chest.
- Inhale and lower your left foot back down to the floor.
- This is one cycle.
- Engage your core muscles to maintain stability and support your lower back. Continue for 15 cycles.

GENERAL TIPS AND COMMON MISTAKES TO AVOID:

- Keep your spine straight and upright throughout the movement to prevent strain on your lower back.
- Ensure your supporting foot remains flat on the floor for stability.

39. STAND UP SIT-DOWNS

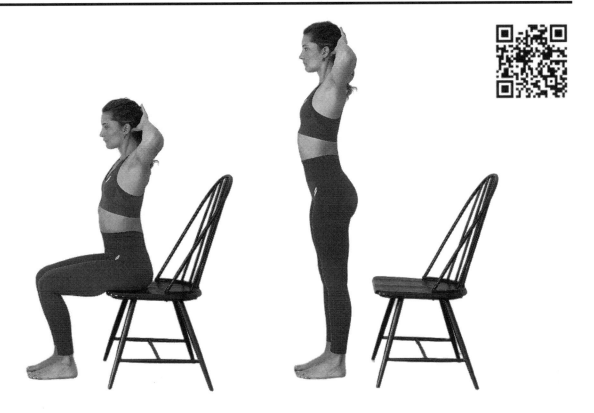

INSTRUCTIONS:

- Begin by sitting toward the front of your chair with your feet hip-width apart and flat on the floor and your hands resting on your thighs.
- Inhale deeply, engage your core muscles, and bring your hands up behind your head, elbows pointing out to the sides.
- Exhale as you lean forward slightly and push through your heels to stand up from the chair.
- Once standing, pause for a moment to ensure your balance.
- Inhale as you slowly lower yourself back down to a seated position, bending your knees and hinging at your hips.
- This is one cycle.
- Repeat the stand-up sit-down motion for 10 cycles.

GENERAL TIPS AND COMMON MISTAKES TO AVOID:

- Ensure that your body remains aligned throughout the exercise. Avoid leaning too far forward when standing up and too far backward when sitting down. This can affect your balance and reduce the effectiveness of the exercise. Keep your head, shoulders, hips, and feet in line with each other, maintaining a straight and upright posture.

40. TOE TOUCH AND REACH

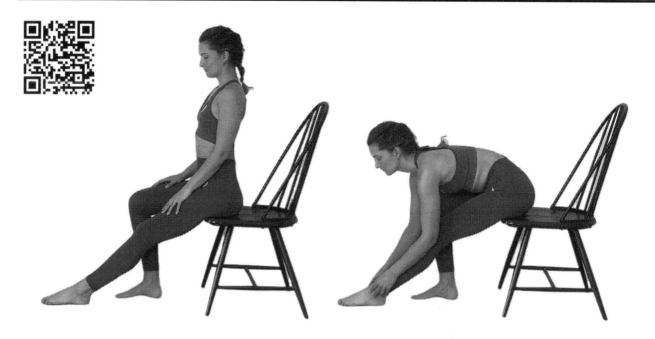

INSTRUCTIONS:

- Sit tall in your chair with your feet flat on the floor and your hands resting on your thighs.
- Inhale deeply, lengthen your spine and straighten your left leg straight out in front of you, feet flat on the floor.
- Exhale as you hinge forward at your hips, reaching your hands towards your toes or the floor.
- Keep your back straight and your chest lifted as you fold forward.
- Inhale and sit back up, bringing your left leg to a bent neutral position.
- On your next inhale, lengthen your spine and straighten your right leg out in front of you, feet flat on the floor.
- Exhale as you hinge forward at your hips, reaching your hands towards your toes or the floor.
- Inhale and return to an upright seated position.
- This is one cycle.
- Continue flowing between left and right toe touches for 8 cycles.

GENERAL TIPS AND COMMON MISTAKES TO AVOID:

- Coordinate the movement with your breath.
- Slow down your breath and movement to flow through the cycle smoothly.
- Avoid rounding the back. Aim for your tummy to touch your thighs before your head touches your legs as you reach forward.

41. LIFT AND KICK

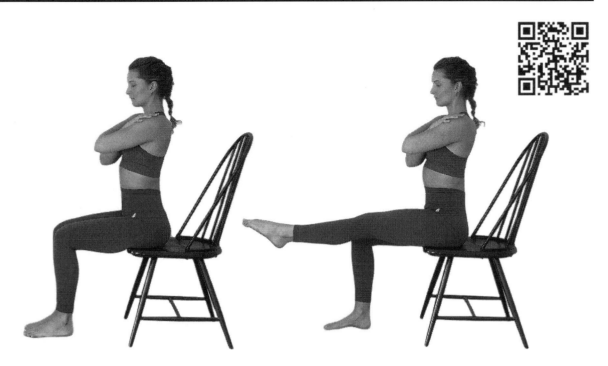

INSTRUCTIONS:

- Sit toward the front of your chair with your feet flat on the floor and your arms crossed on your chest, touching opposite shoulders.
- Inhale deeply and engage your core muscles.
- Exhale as you lift your right leg off the floor, extending it straight out in front of you.
- Inhale to lower your right leg back down to the floor.
- Exhale as you lift your left leg off the floor, extending it straight out in front of you.
- Inhale to lower your left leg back down to the floor.
- This is one cycle.
- Complete 8 cycles.

GENERAL TIPS AND COMMON MISTAKES TO AVOID:

- Coordinate the movement with your breath.
- Slow down your breath and movement to flow through the cycle smoothly.

42. SEATED CROSS PUNCHES

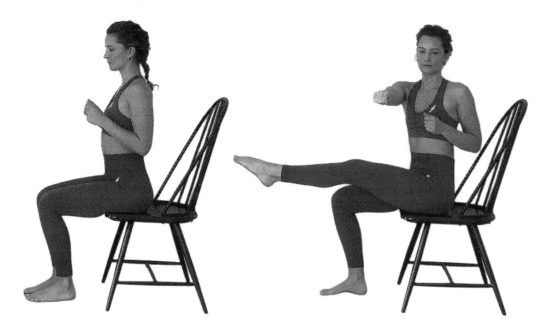

INSTRUCTIONS:

- Sit tall in your chair with your feet flat on the floor and your hands relaxed by your sides.
- Inhale deeply and engage your core muscles.
- Exhale as you twist your torso to the right, bringing your left fist across your body to punch toward the right side while lifting your right leg straight out in front of you.
- Inhale to return to the center.
- Exhale as you twist your torso to the left, bringing your right fist across your body to punch toward the left side while lifting your left leg straight out in front of you.
- This is one cycle.
- Continue for 10 breath cycles.

GENERAL TIPS AND COMMON MISTAKES TO AVOID:

- Ensure your hips remain stable and facing forward; don't let them twist.
- Don't overextend your arm; keep a slight bend in the elbow.
- Keep the punching fist in line with your shoulder. Avoid punching too high or too low.

43. SEATED UPPERCUTS

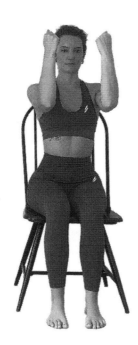 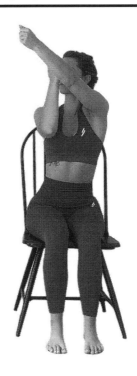

INSTRUCTIONS:

- Sit comfortably in your chair with your feet flat on the floor and your spine tall.
- Engage your core muscles by drawing your navel towards your spine.
- Bring your fists up towards your shoulders, keeping your elbows bent at about a 90-degree angle. Your fists should be in front of your chest, palms facing each other. This is your starting position.
- As you exhale, extend your right arm forward and slightly upward in a diagonal motion, as if you were punching toward the ceiling at a 45-degree angle.
- At the same time, twist your torso to the left, engaging your oblique muscles.
- Inhale as you return your right fist back to the starting position.
- Exhale and extend your left arm forward and slightly upward in a diagonal motion, as if you were punching toward the ceiling at a 45-degree angle.
- At the same time, twist your torso to the right, engaging your oblique muscles.
- Inhale as you return your right fist back to the starting position.
- This is one cycle.
- Repeat this movement for 10 cycles.

GENERAL TIPS AND COMMON MISTAKES TO AVOID:

- Avoid allowing your wrists to collapse or overextend. Keep them in line with your lower arms.
- Ensure your hips remain stable and facing forward; Keep both sit bones in contact with the chair throughout the exercise.

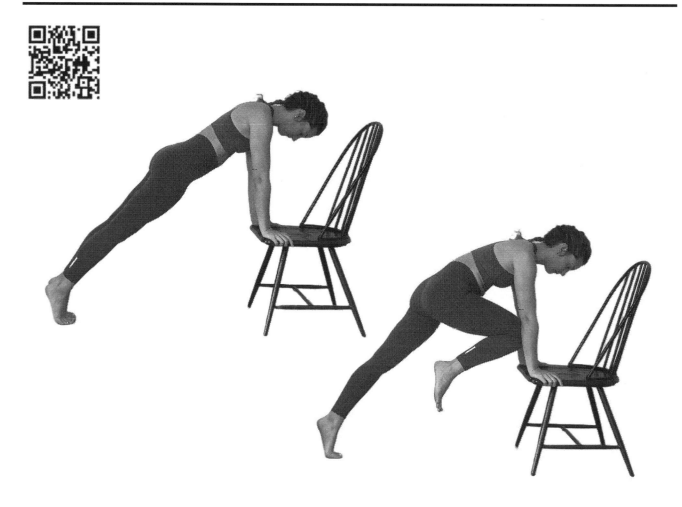

INSTRUCTIONS:

- Start by placing your hands on the seat of the chair, shoulder-width apart, with your arms fully extended.

- Step back into a plank position, with your body forming a straight line from your head to your heels.

- Engage your core muscles to stabilize your body.

- Begin by bringing your right knee towards your chest, then quickly switch legs, bringing your left knee towards your chest while extending your right leg back.

- Continue alternating between bringing your knees towards your chest in a running motion, inhaling on every third movement, and exhaling through the remaining movements.

- Keep a steady rhythm, aiming to continue your chair-assisted mountain climbers for up to 30 seconds.

GENERAL TIPS AND COMMON MISTAKES TO AVOID:

- Ensure your shoulders stay directly above your hands on the chair to maintain stability. Do not allow the chair to slide away from you.

- Roll the shoulders back and down and keep them away from the ears.

- Always extend the legs back to the starting position instead of allowing them to step closer to the chair.

45. CHAIR-ASSISTED SEATED PUSH-UPS

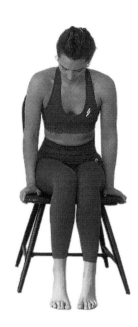 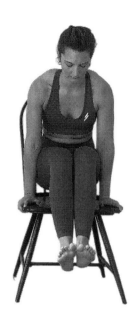

INSTRUCTIONS:

- Sit on the edge of the chair with your hands placed on the seat beside your hips, fingers pointing forward.
- Keep your core engaged and your spine in a straight line from your head to your tailbone.
- Inhale as you straighten your elbows, lifting your body up and your buttocks away from the chair.
- If you can, lift your feet off the floor too.
- Hold this position, focusing on your breath for up to 10 seconds.

GENERAL TIPS AND COMMON MISTAKES TO AVOID:

- Maintain control during this exercise, especially when exiting the pose. Avoid sudden movement or dropping your body on the chair as this may cause injury. Slowly lower your buttocks back on the chair.
- Keep elbows close to your body. Grip the seat of the chair for additional support if necessary.

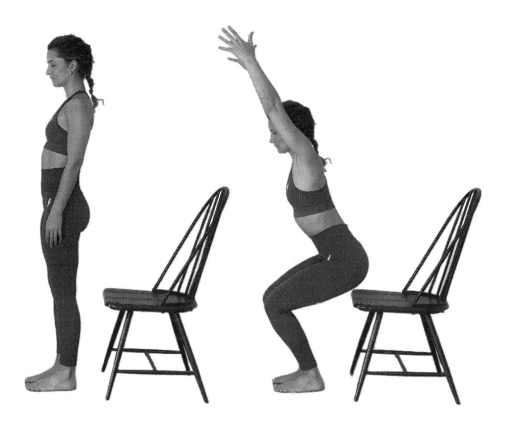

INSTRUCTIONS:

- Stand in front of the chair with your feet hip-width apart.
- Inhale as you raise your arms overhead, palms facing each other or touching.
- Exhale as you bend your knees and lower your hips back as if you were sitting in a chair, while simultaneously reaching your buttocks back towards the chair.
- Keep your chest lifted and your weight in your heels.
- Lower down until your thighs are parallel to the floor or as far as is comfortable for you.
- Hold the elevated chair pose for 10 seconds.
- To come out of the pose, inhale as you straighten your legs and lift your torso back up to standing.

GENERAL TIPS AND COMMON MISTAKES TO AVOID:

- Ensure that the weight is shifted towards the heels in the pose.
- You should "sit" back far enough such that you can see your toes when directing your eyes downwards.

COOLING DOWN

Just as a fire needs a gradual reduction to return to calm embers, so too does your body require a focused cool-down to fully reintegrate after each chair yoga session. Here you will find stretches and breathing sequences that allow your system to transition out of its heightened fat-burning and muscle-building state by regulating your heart rate and easing you back into a state of focused relaxation. Honor these cool-down practices to avoid abruptly short-circuiting your body's physiological cycles. Proper recovery today enhances strength and flexibility for your future training.

47. FULL CACTUS FLOW

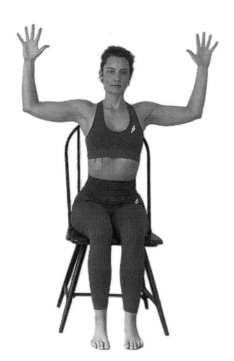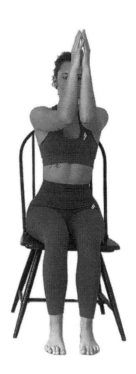

INSTRUCTIONS:

- Sit with your feet hip-width apart and your arms extended out to the sides at shoulder height.
- Bend your elbows to 90 degrees, creating a cactus shape with your arms.
- Exhale and bring your arms together in front of your face, bringing your elbows and palms together.
- Inhale deeply, open your arms out to the sides, and relax your shoulders away from your ears and your chest open.
- This is one cycle.
- Continue this movement for 8 cycles.

GENERAL TIPS AND COMMON MISTAKES TO AVOID:

- Coordinate the movement with your breath.
- Slow down your breath and movement to flow through the cycle smoothly.
- Keep the upper arms parallel to the floor throughout this exercise.

48. HALF-SUN SALUTATION

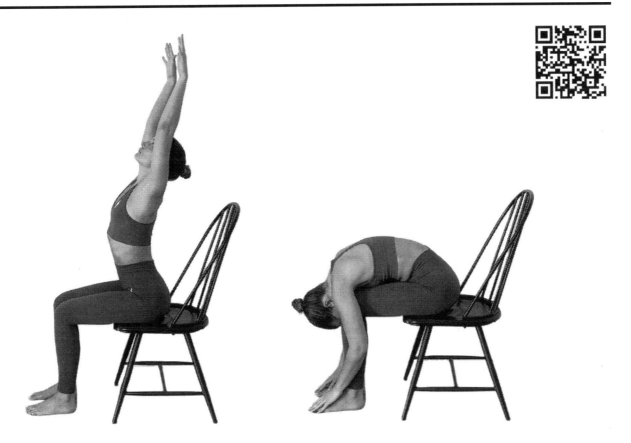

INSTRUCTIONS:

- Sit on the edge of the chair with your feet flat on the floor and your hands resting on your knees.
- Inhale deeply and reach your arms up towards the ceiling, keeping them parallel to each other and shoulder-width apart. If it's comfortable, you can bring your palms together in a prayer position overhead.
- Exhale and hinge at your hips and slowly lower your torso towards your thighs. Let your arms come down towards the floor. Allow your head to hang heavy and relax your neck.
- Inhale and lengthen your spine by lifting your torso slightly, bringing your hands back to your thighs or knees. Keep your back flat and gaze forward.
- Exhale as you slowly bring your torso upright and come back to the starting position.
- This is one cycle.
- Complete for 8 cycles.

GENERAL TIPS AND COMMON MISTAKES TO AVOID:

- Coordinate the movement with your breath.
- Slow down your breath and movement to flow through the cycle smoothly.
- Avoid straining your neck by keeping it in line with your spine. Don't crank your head forward or tilt it too far back.

49. FIVE-POINT STAR

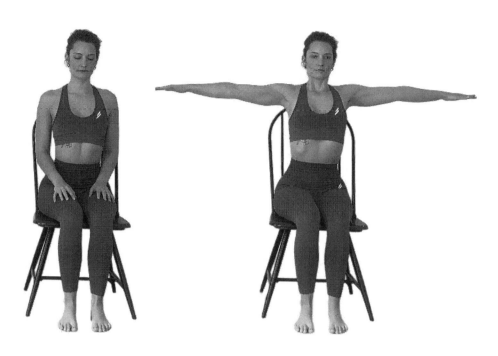

INSTRUCTIONS:

- Sit comfortably in your chair with your feet flat on the floor and your hands resting on your thighs.
- Inhale deeply and raise your arms out to the sides at shoulder height, palms facing down.
- Spread your fingers wide, as if you're reaching towards the walls on either side of you.
- Lift your chest and gaze upwards.
- Hold the five-point star pose for up to 15 seconds, breathing deeply and feeling the stretch through your chest and shoulders.

GENERAL TIPS AND COMMON MISTAKES TO AVOID:

- Be mindful not to overarch your lower back. Engage your core muscles to support your spine and prevent excessive arching.
- Keep your neck in a neutral position and avoid tilting it back excessively. Your gaze can be straight ahead or slightly upward.

50. DOWNWARD DOG

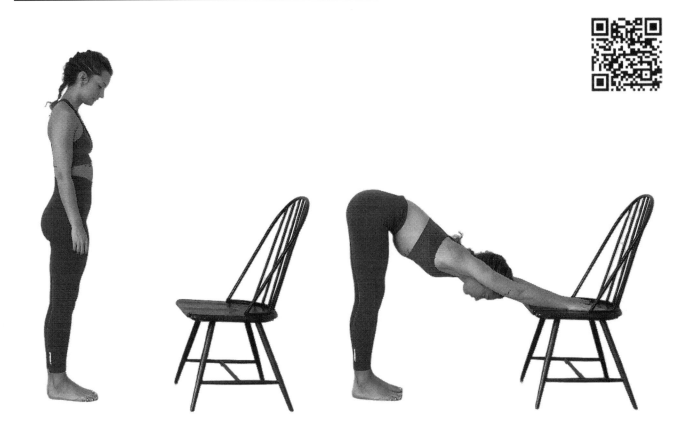

INSTRUCTIONS:

- Stand in front of your chair with your feet flat on the floor.
- Place your hands on the seat of the chair, shoulder-width apart.
- Walk your feet back while ensuring they stay directly below your hips until your body forms a diagonal line from your hands to your hips.
- Press your hands firmly into the chair seat and engage your core muscles.
- Hold the downward dog position for 20-30 seconds, breathing deeply and feeling the stretch through your arms, shoulders, and back.

GENERAL TIPS AND COMMON MISTAKES TO AVOID:

- For a beginner-friendly modification, place your hands on the backrest of the chair instead. Walk your feet back until the upper body is parallel to the floor.
- Aim to lengthen your spine from your tailbone to the crown of your head by bringing your head between your straightened arms.

51. CHILD'S POSE

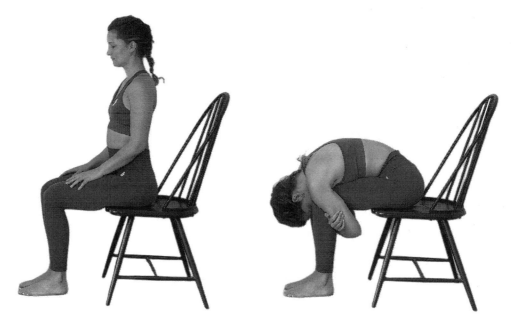

INSTRUCTIONS:

- Sit comfortably in your chair with your feet flat on the floor and your knees bent.
- Lower your torso forward, bringing your chest towards your thighs.
- Rest your forehead on your folded arms or on your knees.
- Allow your chest to sink towards your thighs and feel the stretch through your back and shoulders.
- Wrap your hands around the bottom of your thighs in a hugging position.
- Hold the seated child's pose for up to 15 seconds, breathing deeply and surrendering to the stretch.

GENERAL TIPS AND COMMON MISTAKES TO AVOID:

- Use props as necessary. If your torso does not rest on the thighs comfortably, place a bolster/pillow/folded blanket over your lap and rest your head on that instead.

52. CAT POSE

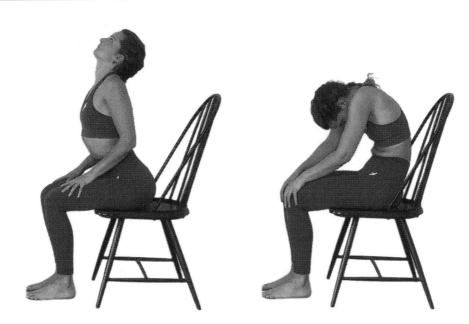

INSTRUCTIONS:

- Sit towards the front edge of your chair with your feet flat on the floor and your hands resting on your thighs.
- Inhale deeply and arch your back, lifting your chest and gazing straight forward.
- Exhale as you round your back, tucking your chin towards your chest and drawing your navel towards your spine.
- This is one cycle.
- Continue flowing between cat and cow poses, moving with your breath and feeling the stretch through your spine for 5 full cycles.

GENERAL TIPS AND COMMON MISTAKES TO AVOID:

- Coordinate the movement with your breath.
- Slow down your breath and movement to flow through the cycle smoothly.

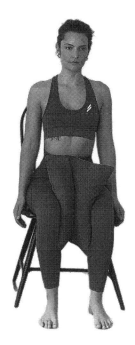
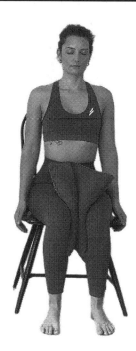

You will need a cushion, a rolled-up towel, or a soft ball for this pose.

INSTRUCTIONS:

- Sit up straight in your chair with your feet flat on the floor and your spine tall.
- Place your cushion, rolled-up towel, or soft ball between your knees.
- Drop your arms down to your sides, palms facing toward the chair.
- Inhale and gently squeeze your knees.
- Exhale and release the squeeze without dropping the ball/towel/cushion. This is one cycle.
- Squeeze and release for 10 full cycles.

GENERAL TIPS AND COMMON MISTAKES TO AVOID:

- Keep your facial muscles relaxed and your jaw unclenched.
- Keep your hips stable and level throughout the movement. Avoid tilting or rocking your pelvis from side to side.
- Keep the soles of both feet in the same position on the floor throughout the movement. Avoid moving the feet closer or further.

CHAPTER 3:
INTEGRATING BREATHWORK INTO CHAIR YOGA

This chapter lays the essential groundwork for a safe and effective chair yoga practice. It begins by guiding you through various yogic breathing exercises to achieve mind-body synergy and energize the postures. You'll then flow through gentle warm-up movements to prepare the body while learning the importance of proper alignment.

Mastering these fundamental breathwork techniques, preparatory sequences, and postural principles is crucial for creating a holistic chair yoga practice. When we approach our workouts with patience and curiosity we can build upon a stable foundation that nurtures and encourages further development and ultimately healthy weight loss.

BREATHING TECHNIQUES

The key to unlocking the profound potential of any yogic practice is the masterful regulation of your breath or pranayama. Breath is the essential force that animates you physically, calms your spirit, and energizes you through your chair yoga practice. In chair yoga, conscious breathwork serves as the vital anchor that roots your being in the present moment while providing a meditative stream upon your mindful movements to flow upon.

Various time-honored breathing techniques are woven into this inclusive discipline, each offering unique benefits for relaxation, focus, mindfulness, and overall well-being. Let us explore three of the core pranayama practices.

The most elemental of all respiration patterns, this technique calls you to concentrate on lowering your breath fully into the belly region with each inhalation. As you draw air in through the nostrils, feel your abdomen expand like a rising bellow. Then as you exhale through softly parted lips, consciously expel all air from your lungs while feeling your belly soften and hollow inward. This rhythmic pattern releases tensions held in the viscera while bathing your cells in rejuvenating oxygen—promoting a state of profound relaxation.

Here you will match your inhalation and exhalation for an equal duration, such as breathing in through the nose for four seconds and then breathing out through the nose for four seconds. This harmonization of the inflow and outflow of your breath fosters a sense of internal balance and equilibrium. As you match the cyclical rhythm, you may find an organic slowing down of your breath rate and heart rate—getting you settled into a zone of calmness and present-moment awareness.

- Sit in a comfortable position on your chair with your feet flat on the ground.
- Ensure your spine is straight and your shoulders are relaxed.
- Close your eyes to help focus inward.
- Take a few natural breaths to settle into your position and become aware of your breathing.
- Inhale slowly through your nose while counting to four (you can adjust this count if it feels too long or too short).
- Hold your breath for a brief moment at the top of your inhale.
- Exhale slowly through your nose (or mouth if you prefer) while counting to four, matching the length of your inhale.
- Try to make the exhale smooth and controlled.
- Continue to inhale for the count of four and exhale for the count of four.
- Maintain the same count for each inhale and exhale to keep the breath equal.
- If four counts feel too short or too long, adjust the count to a number that feels comfortable for you (e.g., counting to three or five).
- Keep your mind focused on the breath and the counting.
- If your mind wanders, gently bring it back to the breath and the count.
- Practice this breathing technique for up to a minute, gradually increasing the duration as you become more accustomed to the practice.
- When you are ready to end the practice, take a few normal breaths.
- Open your eyes slowly and take a moment to notice how you feel.

Generating a soft sonic vibration with each breath cycle, ujjayi pranayama is often referred to as the "ocean breath" due to its soothing, wave-like rhythm. To experience this, partially constrict your throat to create gentle friction against the air stream and your breathing makes a rushing noise almost like a snore. Regulate the breath so that each inhalation and exhalation produces a whispering, oceanic whisper. This focus-enhancing breath stimulates internal heat while cultivating profound concentration and meditative immersion in your practice.

- Sit on your chair with your feet flat on the ground.
- Ensure your spine is straight and your shoulders are relaxed.
- Close your eyes to help focus inward.
- Start by taking a few natural breaths to settle into your position and become aware of your breathing.
- Inhale deeply through your mouth.
- Exhale through your mouth, creating a "ha" sound, as if you were fogging up a mirror.
- On your next exhale, create the same "ha" sound but with your mouth closed. This will cause a slight constriction at the back of your throat, producing a soft, whispering sound.
- Inhale through your nose while maintaining the slight constriction in your throat. The breath should make a gentle, ocean-like sound.
- Exhale through your nose with the same throat constriction, ensuring the exhale is smooth and controlled.
- Continue to inhale and exhale through your nose, maintaining the soft, whispering sound.
- Focus on the sound of your breath and the sensation of the air moving through your throat.
- Aim for a steady, even rhythm in your breathing. The length of the inhale and exhale should be approximately equal.
- If it helps, you can count to four on the inhale and to four on the exhale, similar to Equal Ratio Breathing.
- Continue Ujjayi Breath for up to a minute.
- Gradually increase the duration of your practice as you become more accustomed to the technique.
- When you are ready to end the practice, release the constriction in your throat and take a few normal breaths.
- Open your eyes slowly and take a moment to notice how you feel.

PROPER POSTURE AND ALIGNMENT

While the guided instructions and breathwork techniques lay the physical and metaphysical foundations of your yoga practice, it is through finding alignment within your own body that you can truly gain the transformative capacity of each yoga pose. Proper positioning and adjustment of the anatomy is therefore an indispensable component to be mastered in this chapter.

The spinal column is arguably the most important part of your body; it is around which all other alignments radiate. When you sit upon your chair, imagine a thread pulling the crown of your head upwards as your tailbone anchors down on the chair seat. Maintain this spinal extension by engaging the deep abdominal muscles to provide pyramid-like support as you draw your shoulder blades backward and your front body broadens across your chest.

From this central axis, consciously distribute your weight equally on the two sitting bones you are rooting down through. See if you can align your ears directly over your shoulders, the shoulders over the hips in one seamless plumbline of integrity. Relax your lower body and bring your knees and feet to point directly forward. This total-body alignment is the very embodiment of seated poise and vitality.

To amplify the flow of somatic energies, allow your facial muscles to soften and unfurl. Release any unconscious gripping or clenching of the jaw muscles. Smoothen the forehead and allow your eyes to gaze tenderly ahead without strain. Each ensuing posture will emerge as a natural extension and variation from this position of noble repose.

Remind yourself of these alignment principles frequently and you will find an upright stability that allows you to safely and confidently explore each chair yoga pose. You can also always return to this starting seated position whenever you need to recenter yourself or take a break during your practice.

CHAPTER 4:
WORKOUT ROUTINES

The Full-Body Focus routines enhance flexibility in the shoulders, spine, and hips while building strength and improving overall posture. The accessible movements improve blood circulation and promote relaxation, effectively reducing stress and anxiety, making this routine a holistic approach to enhancing both physical and mental well-being.

Muscle-toning Focus routines offer a comprehensive approach to enhancing muscle strength and overall fitness. These routines target various muscle groups, improving tone and endurance in the arms, legs, and core. They build strength and stability, while still working on flexibility and fostering relaxation.

Fat Burning Focus routines are designed to effectively boost metabolism and promote weight loss. These routines incorporate dynamic movements to increase heart rate and burn calories. Warm-ups prepare the body for exercise, while cool-downs aid in recovery and flexibility. By combining cardio, strength, and flexibility elements, these routines provide a balanced and effective approach to fat-burning and overall fitness.

Side Stretches Focus routines, featuring targeted warm-ups, main exercises, and cool-downs, are crafted to enhance flexibility and strength along the sides of the body. These routines include dynamic stretches and movements which effectively lengthen and tone the lateral muscles. Warm-ups prepare the body by loosening tight muscles, while cool-downs ensure a gentle return to rest and promote overall relaxation. By focusing on lateral flexibility and strength, these routines provide a comprehensive approach to improving range of motion and muscular balance.

Restorative practices offer a gentle and nurturing approach to yoga, prioritizing relaxation and rejuvenation. The objective is to deeply relax into each pose, promoting physical and mental restoration while fostering a sense of release and surrender. By emphasizing extended holds and mindful breathing, these practices facilitate stress relief, improved flexibility, and a heightened sense of well-being, making them ideal for anyone seeking deep relaxation and renewal.

Comprehensive practices: These comprehensive chair yoga routines offer a holistic approach to physical and mental well-being, catering to individuals of all fitness levels. The routines encompass a range of seated poses and gentle movements designed to improve flexibility, strength, and relaxation. Whether seeking gentle stretching or a more dynamic workout, these chair yoga routines provide a versatile and accessible option for enhancing overall health and vitality.

WORK OUT OFFLINE

Below you will find each routine explained in step-by-step and video formats. These routines are broken down not just in step-by-step instructions but also include an illustration and a QR code for you to scan.

Scanning this code will direct you to a short video clip of the exercise so that you can complete the routine with proper posture, alignment, and breathwork.

Additionally, keep in mind that you have access to a free gift that includes a file of all of the routines in video format to download to your computer. This way, you won't need to scan each routine individually. Rather, you can train offline, wherever you are without the need for wifi. To access your gift, scan the QR code provided in the introduction of this book.

FULL-BODY FOCUS A

1. Warm-up: Seated Cat-Cow Stretch (10 repetitions)

2. Main poses: Prayer pose (20 seconds), Warrior I (20 seconds on each side), Boat pose (10 seconds)

3. Cool-down: Child's pose (15 seconds)

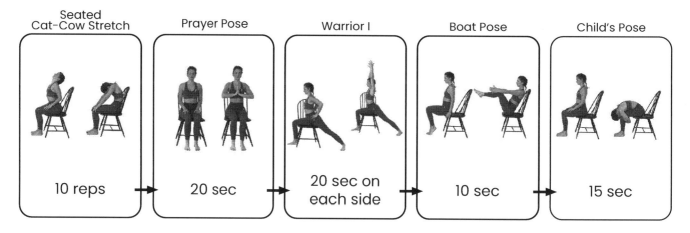

Seated Cat-Cow Stretch	Prayer Pose	Warrior I	Boat Pose	Child's Pose
10 reps	20 sec	20 sec on each side	10 sec	15 sec

FULL-BODY FOCUS B

1. Warm-up: Neck Rolls (10 circles in each direction)

2. Main poses: Cobra (20 seconds), Deep side stretch (10 seconds on each side), Single-leg forward bend (10 seconds on each side)

3. Cool-down: Full Cactus flow (8 cycles)

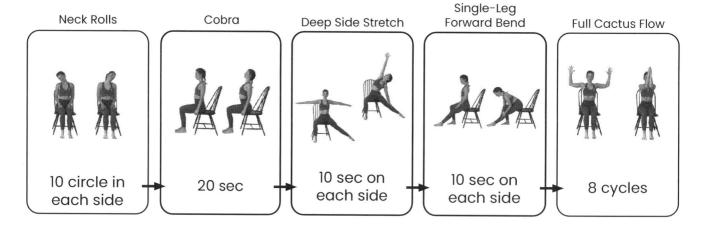

Neck Rolls	Cobra	Deep Side Stretch	Single-Leg Forward Bend	Full Cactus Flow
10 circle in each side	20 sec	10 sec on each side	10 sec on each side	8 cycles

FULL-BODY FOCUS C

1. Warm-up: Shoulder Rolls (10 circles in each direction)

2. Main poses: Side twist (10 seconds on each side), High lunge (10 seconds on each side), Pigeon pose (10 seconds on each side)

3. Cool-down: Downward dog (30 seconds)

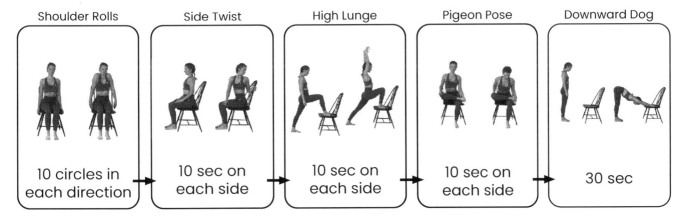

Shoulder Rolls	Side Twist	High Lunge	Pigeon Pose	Downward Dog
10 circles in each direction	10 sec on each side	10 sec on each side	10 sec on each side	30 sec

MUSCLE-TONING FOCUS A

1. Warm-up: Wrist Circles (10 circles in each direction)

2. Main exercises: Chair squats (15 repetitions), Tricep dips (10 cycles), Seated leg raises (10 repetitions)

3. Cool-down: Five-Pointed Star (15 seconds)

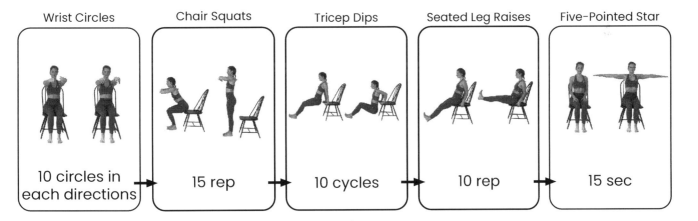

Wrist Circles	Chair Squats	Tricep Dips	Seated Leg Raises	Five-Pointed Star
10 circles in each directions	15 rep	10 cycles	10 rep	15 sec

MUSCLE-TONING FOCUS B

1. Warm-up: Ankle Circles (10 circles in each direction)

2. Main exercises: Calf raises (15 repetitions), Toe taps (15 repetitions), Seated push-ups (10 seconds)

3. Cool-down: Cat pose (5 cycles)

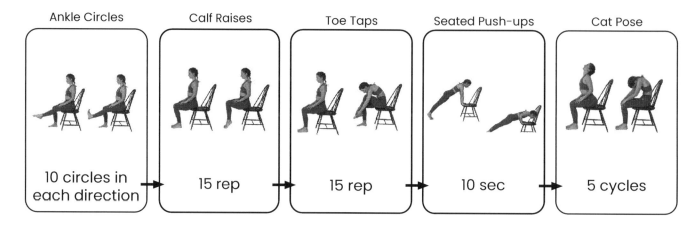

Ankle Circles	Calf Raises	Toe Taps	Seated Push-ups	Cat Pose
10 circles in each direction	15 rep	15 rep	10 sec	5 cycles

MUSCLE-TONING FOCUS C

1. Warm-up: Seated Forward Fold (20 seconds)

2. Main exercises: Knee to nose (10 seconds on each side), Mountain pose (10 cycles), Single-leg calf raises (15 repetitions)

3. Cool-down: Full Cactus flow (8 cycles)

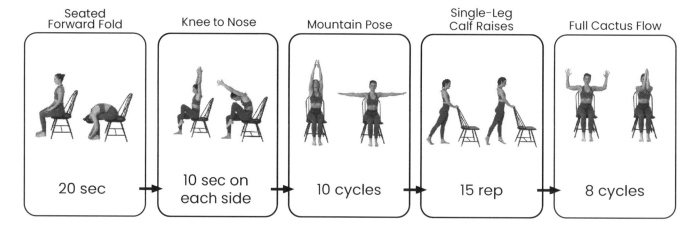

Seated Forward Fold	Knee to Nose	Mountain Pose	Single-Leg Calf Raises	Full Cactus Flow
20 sec	10 sec on each side	10 cycles	15 rep	8 cycles

FAT-BURNING FOCUS A

1. Warm-up: Seated Cat-Cow Stretch (10 repetitions)

2. Main exercises: Seated marching (15 cycles), Toe touch and reach (8 cycles), Elevated chair pose (10 seconds)

3. Cool-down: High Lunge stretch (10 seconds on each side)

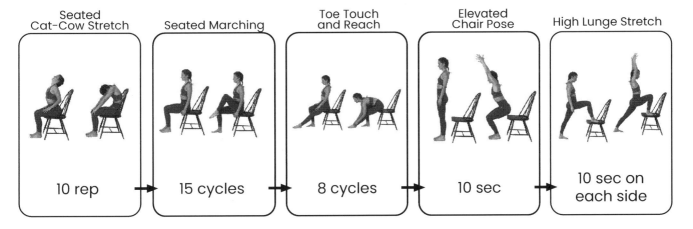

Seated Cat-Cow Stretch	Seated Marching	Toe Touch and Reach	Elevated Chair Pose	High Lunge Stretch
10 rep	15 cycles	8 cycles	10 sec	10 sec on each side

FAT-BURNING FOCUS B

1. Warm-up: Shoulder Rolls (10 circles in each direction)

2. Main exercises: Stand-up sit-downs (10 cycles), Seated cross punches (10 cycles), Chair-assisted mountain climbers (30 seconds)

3. Cool-down: Five-point star (15 seconds)

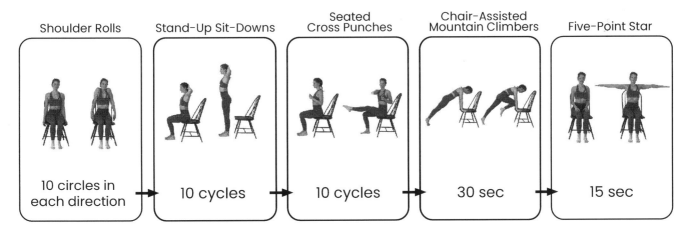

Shoulder Rolls	Stand-Up Sit-Downs	Seated Cross Punches	Chair-Assisted Mountain Climbers	Five-Point Star
10 circles in each direction	10 cycles	10 cycles	30 sec	15 sec

FAT-BURNING FOCUS C

1. Warm-up: Ankle Circles (10 circles in each direction)

2. Main exercises: Lift and kick (8 cycles), Seated uppercuts (10 cycles), Chair-assisted push-ups (2 minutes)

3. Cool-down: Knee Squeeze (10 cycles)

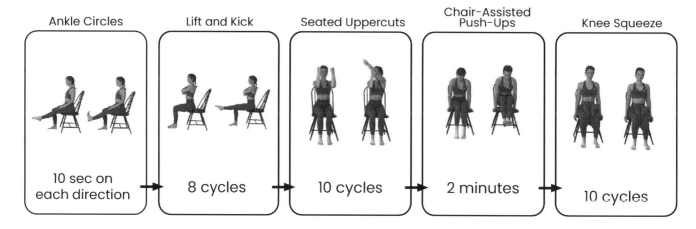

Ankle Circles	Lift and Kick	Seated Uppercuts	Chair-Assisted Push-Ups	Knee Squeeze
10 sec on each direction	8 cycles	10 cycles	2 minutes	10 cycles

SIDE STRETCHES FOCUS A

1. Warm-up: Seated Cat-Cow Stretch (10 repetitions)

2. Main exercises: Sage Pose (30 seconds on each side), Seated Uppercuts (10 cycles), Toe touch and reach (8 cycles)

3. Cool-down: Downward Dog (30 seconds)

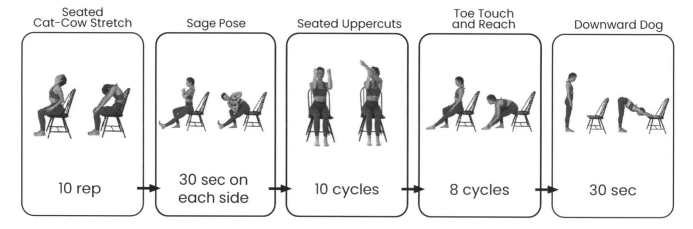

Seated Cat-Cow Stretch	Sage Pose	Seated Uppercuts	Toe Touch and Reach	Downward Dog
10 rep	30 sec on each side	10 cycles	8 cycles	30 sec

SIDE STRETCHES FOCUS B

1. Warm-up: Shoulder Rolls (10 circles in each direction)

2. Main exercises: Side Twist (30 seconds on each side), Deep Side Stretch (10 seconds on each side), Seated Cross Punches (10 cycles)

3. Cool-down: Five-point star (15 seconds)

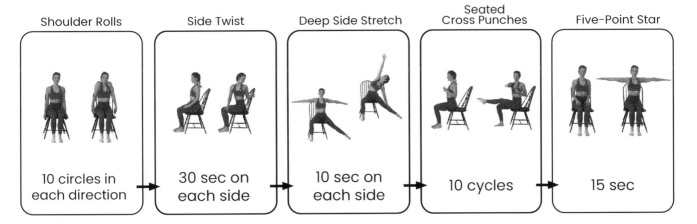

Shoulder Rolls	Side Twist	Deep Side Stretch	Seated Cross Punches	Five-Point Star
10 circles in each direction	30 sec on each side	10 sec on each side	10 cycles	15 sec

SIDE STRETCHES FOCUS C

1. Warm-up: Neck Rolls (10 circles in each direction)

2. Main exercises: Cowface Arms (30 seconds on each side), Revolved Pose (30 seconds on each side), Chair-Assisted Mountain Climbers (30 seconds)

3. Cool-down: Full Cactus Flow (8 cycles)

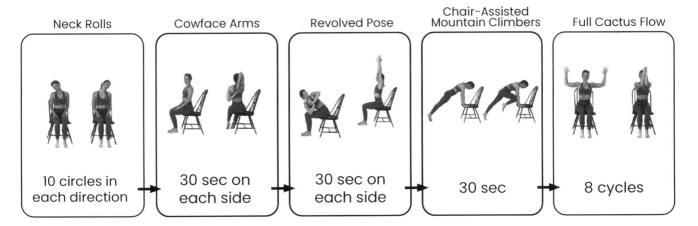

Neck Rolls	Cowface Arms	Revolved Pose	Chair-Assisted Mountain Climbers	Full Cactus Flow
10 circles in each direction	30 sec on each side	30 sec on each side	30 sec	8 cycles

RESTORATIVE A

1. Main exercises: Mountain Pose (one minute), Prayer Pose (one minute), Seated Fold Pose (one minute)

2. Cool-down: Five-point star

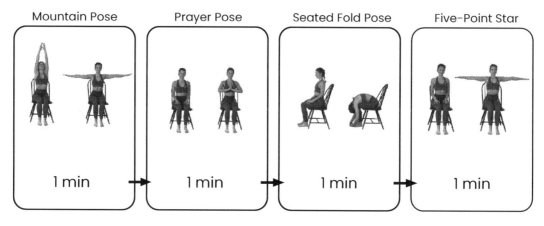

Mountain Pose	Prayer Pose	Seated Fold Pose	Five-Point Star
1 min	1 min	1 min	1 min

RESTORATIVE B

1. Main exercises: Roll-Down, Roll-Up (15 cycles), Cowface Arms (30 seconds on each side), Humble Warrior (30 seconds on each side)

2. Cool-down: Downward Dog (30 seconds up to a minute)

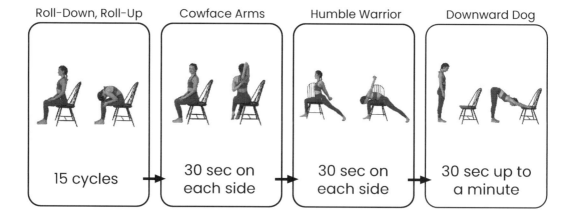

Roll-Down, Roll-Up	Cowface Arms	Humble Warrior	Downward Dog
15 cycles	30 sec on each side	30 sec on each side	30 sec up to a minute

RESTORATIVE C

1. Main exercises: Sun Breath (one minute), Sage Pose (one minute), Pigeon Pose (one minute)

2. Cool-down: Child's Pose (one minute)

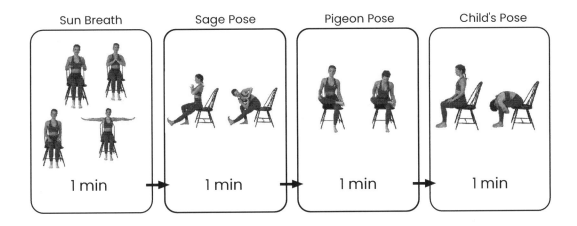

Sun Breath	Sage Pose	Pigeon Pose	Child's Pose
1 min	1 min	1 min	1 min

COMPLETE (SEATED) CHAIR YOGA ROUTINE

1. Warm-up: Shoulder Rolls (10 circles in each direction), Ankle Circles (10 circles in each direction)

2. Main exercises: Hands Up (20 seconds), Cactus Arms (20 seconds), Seated Fold Pose (20 seconds), Cowface Arms (30 seconds on each side), Revolved Pose (30 seconds on each side), Leg Extensions (15 repetitions each side), Calf Raises (15 repetitions), Shuffle Legs (15 repetitions), Foot Flexor (5 repetitions), Toe Taps (15 repetitions)

3. Cool-down: Half-Sun Salutations (8 cycles)

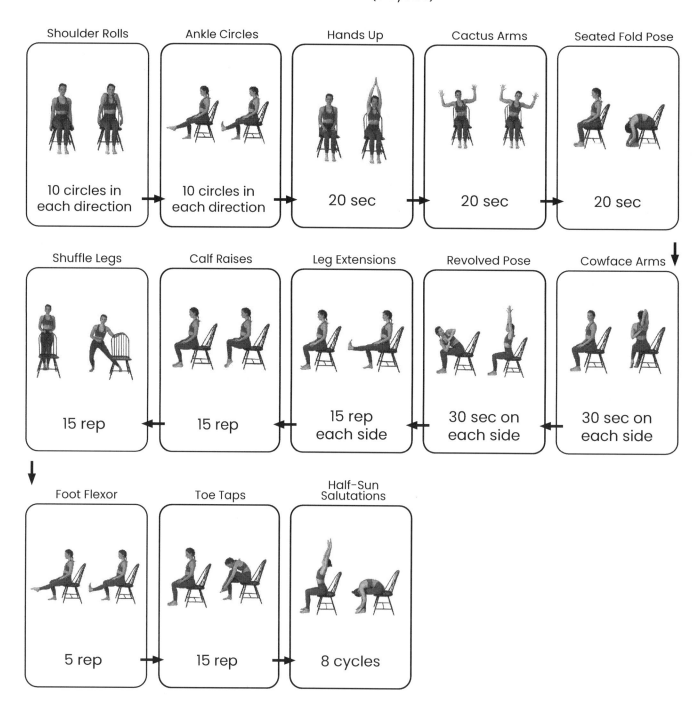

COMPLETE CHAIR YOGA ROUTINE

1. Warm-up: Wrist Circles (10 circles in each direction), Seated Cat-Cow Stretch (10 repetitions)

2. Main exercises: Sun Breath (5 cycles), Side Twist (10 seconds on each side), Low Lunge (10 seconds on each side), Humble Warrior (10 seconds on each side), Chair Push-Ups (10 cycles), Roll-Down, Roll-Up (5 cycles), Sage Pose (30 seconds on each side), Boat Pose (10 seconds), Pigeon Pose (10 seconds on each side)

3. Cool-down: Five-Point Star (15 seconds), Child's Pose (15 seconds to one minute)

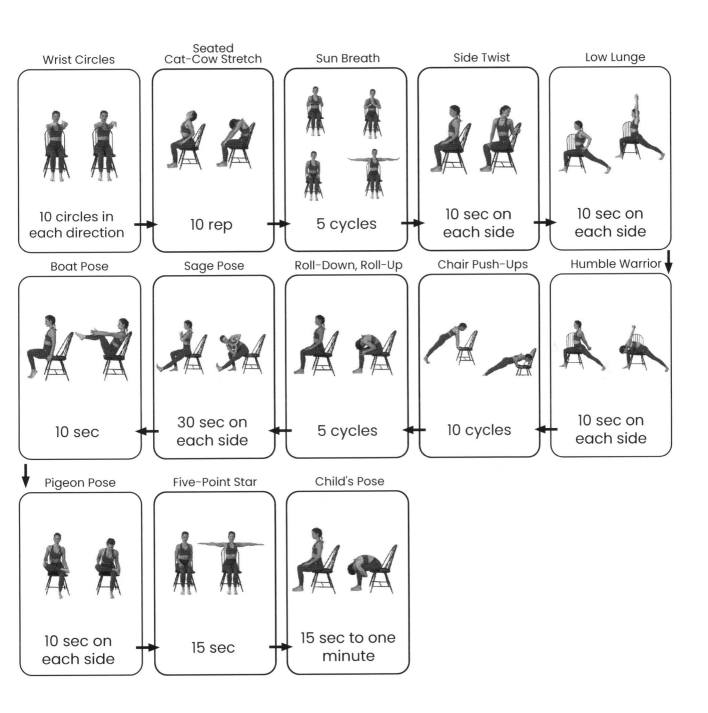

CHAPTER 5:
28-DAY CHALLENGE

The teachings and practices explored thus far have initiated you into the revitalizing world of chair yoga. You now possess a stable foundation in postural alignment, breath work, and the embodiment of adapted asanas. Yet the truest integration arises through sustained devotion over time—a commitment to the heart of this transformative journey—your 28-Day Chair Yoga Challenge is a carefully structured, progressive four-week program facilitating an incremental deepening of your practice.

Each week builds upon the previous, establishing somatic baselines before amplifying the dynamic and static strengthening elements. As the physical intensifies, mindfulness practices temper the steel of the body with the unconditional acceptance of the spirit.

Fully surrender to this immersive progression to organically unite movement with breath, form with energy, becoming one with your body and mind. The culminating synthesis awakens an experience of integrated mastery.

This process demands patience and discipline. There will be days where the postures seem impassable or the mind goes astray. Yet these are precisely the moments of lucid unfolding. By persistently returning to the breath and aligning with the goal, you initiate the necessary shedding of all that impedes your progress.

So approach the 28-Day Challenge with a humble heart and a valiant spirit. Those who weather the tempering storms unveil their innate splendor as radiant, capable beings. You've been granted the tools—now bravely walk the path.

MONITORING YOUR PROGRESS WITH THE FITNESS TRACKER

Below, you will find your complimentary fitness tracker. This useful tool provides you with prompts to maximize your chair yoga workout and monitor your progress as you. Your tracker includes:

- A daily challenge.
- Space to note physical sensations.
- A place to check off each completed day of your challenge.

Remember, you have this fitness tracker included in your gift pack. Print it out, stick it up in your workout area, tick off each day you complete, and use it as a way to celebrate your incredible progress!

Keep in mind that your gift is available to you by scanning the QR code in the introduction of this book.

Welcome to the start of your transformative 28-day chair yoga journey. This first week establishes a solid base for the challenge ahead by introducing foundational routines to be built on week by week. Each day's practice plants seeds of strength and flexibility that will flourish in the coming weeks. Approach these initial routines with an open mind and patience, allowing your body to acclimate to this new, health-promoting rhythm.

DAY 1	DAY 2	DAY 3	DAY 4
Full-Body Focus A	Muscle-Toning Focus A	Fat Burning Focus A	Side Stretches Focus A
pag. 72	pag. 73	pag. 75	pag. 76

DAY 5	DAY 6	DAY 7
Restorative A	Complete (Seated) Chair Yoga Routine	Rest Day
pag. 78	pag. 80	

DAY 1	DAY 2	DAY 3	DAY 4	DAY 5	DAY 6	DAY 7
I BEGIN THE 28-DAY CHAIR YOGA CHALLENGE	A NEW POSTURE I LEARNED TODAY	I'VE COMPLETED ALL THE EXERCISES FROM DAY 3	I DO THE SESSION INCLUDING DEEP AND MINDFUL BREATHING	I SHARE MY CHAIR YOGA EXPERIENCE WITH...	ONE BENEFIT I HAD TODAY	I'VE COMPLETED THE FIRST WEEK OF THE CHALLENGE
☐	☐	☐	☐	☐	☐	☐
I FEEL...	I FEEL...	I FEEL...	I FEEL...	I FEEL...	I FEEL...	I FEEL...

Use the prompts to track your daily exercise and use the blank space to jot down a feeling, your mood, or reflections on your practice.

Don't forget to place an 'X' in each square as you progress!

WEEK 2

As you enter the second week, your commitment is already shaping positive change. The routines now build upon your growing body awareness and stamina. You may notice increased ease in holding poses and deeper breaths. This week's slightly more challenging sequences are designed to further enhance your strength and flexibility. Your determination through the first week has prepared you well - trust in your expanding capabilities.

DAY 8	DAY 9	DAY 10	DAY 11
Full-Body Focus B	Muscle-Toning Focus B	Fat Burning Focus B	Side Stretches Focus B
pag. 72	pag. 74	pag. 75	pag. 77
DAY 12	DAY 13	DAY 14	
Restorative B	Complete (Seated) Chair Yoga Routine	Rest Day	
pag. 78	pag. 80		

DAY 8	DAY 9	DAY 10	DAY 11	DAY 12	DAY 13	DAY 14
A BREATHING TECHNIQUE I PRACTICED TODAY	I'VE PRACTICED CHAIR YOGA FOR 9 CONSECUTIVE DAYS	A POSTURE THAT IS CHALLENGING FOR ME, BUT I WILL CONTINUE PRACTICING TO IMPROVE IT	A NEW POSTURE I LEARNED TODAY	I SHARE MY CHAIR YOGA PROGRESS WITH...	A POSTURE I NOW PERFORM BETTER	I'VE REACHED THE HALFWAY POINT OF THE CHAIR YOGA CHALLENGE
☐	☐	☐	☐	☐	☐	☐
I FEEL...	I FEEL...	I FEEL...	I FEEL...	I FEEL...	I FEEL...	I FEEL...

Use the prompts to track your daily exercise and use the blank space to jot down a feeling, your mood, or reflections on your practice.

Don't forget to place an 'X' in each square as you progress!

Midway through the challenge, you've already accomplished so much. The intensity increases this week, but so does your resilience. If you encounter moments of difficulty, remember how far you've come. Each pose, each breath, is a step toward your goals. Your body is adapting, becoming stronger and more flexible with each practice. Stay focused on the positive changes you're experiencing, both physical and mental.

DAY 15	DAY 16	DAY 17	DAY 18
Full-Body Focus C	Muscle-Toning Focus C	Fat Burning Focus C	Side Stretches Focus C
pag. 73	pag. 74	pag. 76	pag. 77
DAY 19	**DAY 20**	**DAY 21**	
Restorative C	Complete Chair Yoga Routine	Rest Day	
pag. 79	pag. 81		

DAY 15	DAY 16	DAY 17	DAY 18	DAY 19	DAY 20	DAY 21
I PRACTICE CHAIR YOGA FOR 20 UNINTERRUPTED MINUTES	A POSTURE I COULDN'T DO BEFORE	I'VE DID A SESSION OF DEEP AND MINDFUL BREATHING	A POSTURE I NOW PERFORM WITH MORE BALANCE	I'VE REALIZED THAT I HAVE IMPROVED IN...	I'VE INCORPORATED MEDITATION INTO MY DAILY ROUTINE	I'VE COMPLETED 3 WEEKS OF CHAIR YOGA!
☐	☐	☐	☐	☐	☐	☐
I FEEL...	I FEEL...	I FEEL...	I FEEL...	I FEEL...	I FEEL...	I FEEL...

Use the prompts to track your daily exercise and use the blank space to jot down a feeling, your mood, or reflections on your practice.

Don't forget to place an 'X' in each square as you progress!

You're entering the final week of the challenge - the summit is in sight! Reflect on your journey: from those first tentative poses to the confident, mindful practitioner you've become. The strength, flexibility, and calm you've cultivated are now an integral part of you. This week, you get to choose the routine of each weekday. Pick your favorite of the three or one that will push your limits; you know what's best for yourself. Finish strong, knowing that your dedication has laid the groundwork for lasting health and wellness.

DAY 22	DAY 23	DAY 24	DAY 25
Full-Body Focus A, B or C	Muscle-Toning Focus A, B or C	Fat Burning Focus A, B or C	Side Stretches Focus A, B or C
DAY 26	**DAY 27**	**DAY 28**	
Restorative A, B or C	Complete Chair Yoga Routine pag. 81	Rest Day	

DAY 22	DAY 23	DAY 24	DAY 25	DAY 26	DAY 27	DAY 28
A POSTURE I NOW PERFORM BETTER	I JOT DOWN 3 WAYS IN WHICH CHAIR YOGA IS HELPING ME	A POSTURE I CAN NOW HOLD FOR A LONGER TIME	AN IMPROVEMENT I EXPERIENCED TODAY	A POSTURE I CAN NOW DO WITHOUT DISCOMFORT	I'VE DONE A MORE ADVANCED CHAIR YOGA POSES	I'VE SUCCESSFULLY COMPLETED THE 28-DAY CHAIR YOGA CHALLENGE!
☐	☐	☐	☐	☐	☐	☐
I FEEL...	I FEEL...	I FEEL...	I FEEL...	I FEEL...	I FEEL...	I FEEL...

Use the prompts to track your daily exercise and use the blank space to jot down a feeling, your mood, or reflections on your practice.

Don't forget to place an 'X' in each square as you progress!

CHAPTER 6
BEYOND THE CHAIR

As you progress through each day of the 28-Day Chair Yoga Challenge, the teachings and practices you have embraced begin to transform your way of living in a powerful and lasting way. With each passing day, you may find yourself experiencing increased physical vitality, mental clarity, and a deeper understanding of yourself. This journey, however, is just the beginning. Chapter 6 is designed to guide you through the exciting opportunities that await you as you continue to explore and grow in your chair yoga practice.

The path ahead is filled with possibilities for further self-discovery, personal development, and the cultivation of a more balanced, fulfilling life. As you move forward, remember that the skills and insights you have gained during this challenge will serve as a strong foundation for your ongoing journey. Embrace the transformative power of chair yoga and approach each new day with curiosity, openness, and a commitment to nurturing your well-being.

WAYS TO CONTINUE CHAIR YOGA

Establishing a sustainable, long-term chair yoga practice is the first step in integrating these revitalizing techniques into your lifelong health and fitness journey. Now that you've experienced the benefits firsthand, you have the knowledge and understanding to prioritize a committed, consistent practice. But knowledge and understanding are only a part of the equation and you're going to need to sustain your motivation by making chair yoga a regular part of your routine.

This means scheduling dedicated sessions three to four times a week at times that work best with your existing lifestyle so that you don't feel like your chair yoga workouts are a chore.

As you become more comfortable with the foundational poses and sequences, don't be afraid to expand your practice and explore new variations. Each new pose or modification, no matter how small, will help you develop a deeper understanding of your body and its capabilities.

When you feel ready, gradually progress to more advanced postures, the Marichi's Twist and Upward Plank, always listening to your body and moving at a pace that feels safe and comfortable for you.

One of the most powerful aspects of chair yoga is its ability to cultivate mindfulness and meditation through movement. As you continue to refine your breath work, aim to release any tensions or distractions with each exhalation, allowing yourself to be fully present in the moment. Consider incorporating a meditation practice while holding one of your favorite poses, focusing on the connection between your breath, body, and mind. By combining movement and awareness, you can accelerate the integration of your physical and spiritual well-being.

Remember, your chair yoga journey is a personal one, and there is no right or wrong way to progress. Trust your instincts, be patient with yourself, and celebrate the small victories along the way. As you continue to prioritize your practice and explore new dimensions of chair yoga, you'll find that the benefits extend far beyond the physical, enriching your life in countless ways.

PROGRESSIVE PRACTICES

As you advance in your chair yoga journey, incorporating progressive practices can help you continue to challenge yourself, improve your fitness levels, and achieve new milestones. By exploring new techniques and integrating chair yoga with other forms of exercise, you can create a dynamic and engaging practice that supports your weight loss goals and overall well-being.

One way to take your chair yoga practice to the next level is by combining it with other forms of exercise. By integrating chair yoga with strength training, cardiovascular workouts, or Pilates, you can create a well-rounded fitness routine that supports weight loss and overall health.

For example, you might start your workout with a few minutes of gentle chair yoga to warm up your body and focus your mind. Then, move on to a series of strength training exercises using dumbbells or resistance bands, targeting major muscle groups such as your legs, arms, and core. Finish your routine with a few more minutes of chair yoga to cool down, stretch, and promote relaxation.

Alternatively, you might alternate between chair yoga and cardiovascular exercise throughout the week. On days when you practice chair yoga, focus on building flexibility, balance, and mind-body awareness. On alternate days, engage in activities like walking, swimming, or cycling to get your heart rate up and burn additional calories.

Integrating chair yoga with other fitness modalities allows you to create a comprehensive approach to weight loss and wellness that is both effective and enjoyable. This holistic approach not only helps you shed unwanted pounds but also improves your overall fitness level, increases your energy, and promotes a greater sense of well-being.

As you explore these progressive practices, remember to be patient with yourself and celebrate your progress along the way. Each small step forward is a victory, and every challenge overcome is a testament to your dedication and resilience.

In addition to incorporating props and integrating other fitness modalities, consider expanding your chair yoga practice by exploring new poses and sequences. As you become more comfortable with the foundational poses, challenge yourself to try variations or advanced modifications that target different muscle groups or require greater balance and coordination.

For example, if you've mastered the seated forward bend, try adding a twist to the pose to engage your obliques and stimulate digestion. Or, if you're comfortable with the seated mountain pose, explore variations like the seated goddess pose or the seated warrior pose to build strength and confidence.

As you progress in your practice, you may also find it helpful to attend chair yoga classes or workshops led by experienced instructors. These sessions can provide valuable guidance, support, and inspiration, helping you refine your technique, deepen your understanding of the practice, and connect with a community of like-minded individuals.

VINYASA TO ADVANCE YOUR CHAIR YOGA PRACTICE

As you continue to explore and deepen your chair yoga practice, incorporating vinyasa sequences can be a powerful way to challenge yourself, build strength and flexibility, and elevate your overall fitness level. Vinyasa, which means "to place in a special way" in Sanskrit, refers to the flowing, dynamic movements that link one pose to the next in synchronization with the breath.

In the context of chair yoga, vinyasa sequences involve moving seamlessly from one seated or standing pose to another, using the chair for support and stability as needed. By connecting each movement with an inhalation or exhalation, you create a rhythmic, meditative flow that engages your entire body and mind.

One example of a chair yoga vinyasa sequence might begin with seated cat-cow tilts to warm up the spine, followed by a series of seated sun salutations to build heat and energy. From there, you might flow into poses like seated forward bends, twists, and lateral stretches, using the breath to guide your movements and deepen your stretches.

As you become more comfortable with the basic vinyasa sequences, you can explore more advanced variations that incorporate standing poses, balancing postures, and dynamic transitions. For example, you might move from a seated forward bend into a standing forward fold, using the chair for support as you rise up and fold down.

Another advanced vinyasa sequence might involve flowing from a seated twist into a standing warrior pose, using the chair to help you balance as you open your hips and chest. From there, you might transition into a standing side angle pose, using the chair to deepen the stretch in your side body.

The beauty of chair yoga vinyasa is that it allows you to create a customized, dynamic practice that suits your individual needs and goals. By linking poses together in a continuous flow, you can build cardiovascular endurance, increase your flexibility and range of motion, and strengthen key muscle groups throughout your body.

To get started with chair yoga vinyasa, begin by mastering a few basic sequences that feel comfortable and achievable for your current fitness level. As you gain confidence and strength, gradually incorporate more advanced poses and transitions, always listening to your body and honoring your limits.

Remember to focus on your breath throughout each vinyasa sequence, letting the inhalations and exhalations guide your movements and help you stay present in the moment. If you find yourself struggling to keep up with the flow, simply return to your breath and move at a pace that feels sustainable and nourishing for your body.

In addition to the physical benefits, chair yoga vinyasa can also be a powerful tool for reducing stress, calming the mind, and cultivating a greater sense of inner peace and clarity. By synchronizing your movements with your breath, you create a moving meditation that helps you release tension, quiet mental chatter, and find a sense of grounding and centering.

As you continue to explore and evolve your chair yoga vinyasa practice, be sure to listen to your body and honor your unique needs and limitations. Remember, the goal is not to achieve a perfect pose or sequence but rather to cultivate a sense of awareness, compassion, and joy in your practice.

So, whether you're flowing through a gentle seated sequence or challenging yourself with more advanced standing poses, approach your chair yoga vinyasa with a sense of curiosity, openness, and self-love. With regular practice and patience, you'll soon discover the transformative power of this dynamic, flowing approach to chair yoga.

CONCLUSION

Dear Reader,

If these pages could exhale a culminating breath, it would be one of reverent celebration for the profound journey you have undertaken. For in committing yourself to the sacred teachings and practices contained within this volume, you have activated nothing less than a renewal of your entire mind-body-spirit connection.

Reflect upon where you began—the yearnings that first drew you towards the inclusive discipline of chair yoga. Whether beginner or newly remobilized after injury or age, you boldly opened yourself to an awakening process that has subsequently recharged your very being.

Together, we covered breathing techniques, proper posture, and alignment, as well as more than 50 adapted-for-chair yoga poses. The catalog of asanas, along with the wealth of knowledge within these pages, is specially curated to help you enhance your flexibility, strength, and metabolism which aids natural weight regulation.

But far transcending the physical plane, these somatic practices aim to elevate your mental well-being as well. Do you notice a magnified self-awareness bestowed upon you from the application of mindfulness and meditative teachings? May you continue to mold yourself into a being of poise, clarity, and unshakable centeredness.

I would like to request one humble act in return—that you honor this ineffable transformation by providing an honest review of your experience. Let your inspiring story serve as a beacon for the next wave of seekers. For in sharing your earned wisdom, the perpetual journey continues, rolling eternally upon itself.

Namaste, radiant one. The path forever unfurls.

YOUR FEEDBACK MATTERS: LEAVE A REVIEW AND SHARE YOUR THOUGHTS

We are thrilled that you have chosen to read all the tips and information mentioned in this book as a companion to help you achieve a healthier and fitter body through chair yoga. We hope it brings value, enriches perspectives, and ignites the passion to achieve a more independent life thanks to a body that is comfortable to move around in. We greatly appreciate your support, and we hope you are enjoying your new book.

From Balanced Living Books, we plan to continue providing content that inspires as many people to live physically active and healthy lifestyles, and your opinion matters in this process. If you found this book enjoyable, inspiring, and helpful, kindly consider leaving a review and sharing your thoughts with others by scanning this QR code. Your feedback can make significant differences; both to help people out there discover the valuable benefits of this book and to allow us to continue offering content that resonates with what people need to stay healthy.

Made in United States
Orlando, FL
22 September 2024

51792919R00059